CONFRONTING HEREDITARY BREAST AND OVARIAN CANCER

A JOHNS HOPKINS PRESS HEALTH BOOK

CONFRONTING HEREDITARY BREAST AND OVARIAN CANCER

Identify Your Risk, Understand Your Options, Change Your Destiny

SUE FRIEDMAN, D.V.M.

REBECCA SUTPHEN, M.D.

KATHY STELIGO

Foreword by Mark H. Greene, M.D.

ENDORSED BY
FACING OUR RISK OF CANCER EMPOWERED
(FORCE)

THE JOHNS HOPKINS UNIVERSITY PRESS
Baltimore

© 2012 The Johns Hopkins University Press
All rights reserved. Published 2012
Printed in the United States of America on acid-free paper
9 8 7 6 5 4 3 2 1

The Johns Hopkins University Press
2715 North Charles Street
Baltimore, Maryland 21218-4363
www.press.jhu.edu

A catalog record for this book is available from the British Library.

Special discounts are available for bulk purchases of this book. For more information, please contact Special Sales at 410-516-6936 or specialsales@press.jhu.edu.

The Johns Hopkins University Press uses environmentally friendly book materials, including recycled text paper that is composed of at least 30 percent post-consumer waste, whenever possible.

LIBRARY OF CONGRESS CATALOGING-IN-PUBLICATION DATA

Friedman, Sue.
  Confronting hereditary breast and ovarian cancer : identify your risk, understand your options, change your destiny / Sue Friedman, Rebecca Sutphen, and Kathy Steligo ; foreword by Mark H. Greene.
    p.   cm. — (A Johns Hopkins Press health book)
  Includes bibliographical references and index.
  ISBN-13: 978-1-4214-0407-3 (hardcover : alk. paper)
  ISBN-13: 978-1-4214-0408-0 (pbk. : alk. paper)
  ISBN-10: 1-4214-0407-9 (hardcover : alk. paper)
  ISBN-10: 1-4214-0408-7 (pbk. : alk. paper)
  1. Breast—Cancer—Genetic aspects—Popular works. 2. Breast—Cancer—Risk factors—Popular works. 3. Breast—Cancer—Prevention—Popular works. 4. Ovaries—Cancer—Genetic aspects—Popular works. 5. Ovaries—Cancer—Risk factors—Popular works. 6. Ovaries—Cancer—Prevention—Popular works. I. Sutphen, Rebecca. II. Steligo, Kathy. III. Title.
  RC280.B8F739 2012
  616.99'449042—dc23   2011019918

Contents

FOREWORD *by Mark H. Greene, M.D.* xi

ACKNOWLEDGMENTS xv

INTRODUCTION xvii

PART I. UNDERSTANDING CANCER, GENETICS, AND RISK

CHAPTER 1. Breast and Ovarian Cancer Basics 3

Most Cancers Aren't Hereditary 3

An Introduction to Breast Cancer 4

An Introduction to Ovarian Cancer 8

Other Hereditary Cancers 11

CHAPTER 2. A Peek Inside: Your Genes at Work 14

The Evolution of Genetic Discovery: From Peas to BRCA 14

Your Genetic ABCs . . . and a D 16

Mutations: Spelling Errors in Your DNA Cookbook 18

How Mutations Lead to Cancer 20

What's So Special about BRCA? 22

CHAPTER 3. Defining Risk 25

Making Sense of Statistics 26

Getting Personal: Factors That Modify Your Risk 28

It's a Numbers Game 31

CHAPTER 4. Hereditary Cancer: What's Swimming in Your Gene Pool? 36

Mutations from Mom or Dad 36

Hidden Risk in the Family Tree 37

HBOC and Other Hereditary Cancer Syndromes 38

Plotting Your Genetic Pedigree 42

PART II. ASSESSING YOUR RISK

CHAPTER 5. Genetic Counseling 49

The Value of Counseling 49

What to Expect from the Process 50

Why You Need an Expert to Unravel Your Genetic History 52

Deciding Who Should Test First 54

CHAPTER 6. Genetic Testing: Facing Your Hereditary Horoscope 58

Which Test Is Right for You? 58

Powerful, Yet Imperfect 60

Issues for Survivors and Women in Treatment 61

CHAPTER 7. Decoding Your Test Results 67

Life, Interrupted: It's Positive 67

Good News! You're a True Negative 68

When No Might Mean Maybe 68

Genetic Variants 70

Now What? Implications for You and Your Family 71

PART III. MANAGING YOUR RISK:
YOUR DNA DOESN'T HAVE TO BE YOUR DESTINY

CHAPTER 8. Early Detection Strategies 77

High-Risk Surveillance for Breast Cancer 77

High-Risk Surveillance for Ovarian Cancer 84

Is It Cancer? 88

Screening for Other Hereditary Cancers 90

CHAPTER 9. Chemoprevention 94

Risk-Reducing Medications for Breast Cancer 94
Alternatives under Study 99
Chemoprevention for Ovarian Cancer 103

CHAPTER 10. Mastectomy for Risk Reduction and Treatment 107

Reducing Cancer Risk by Removing the Breasts 107
Skin-Sparing Procedures 110
Treating Breast Cancer with Mastectomy 114
Who Should Perform Your Surgery? 116
Risks and Recovery 116

CHAPTER 11. Reconstruction: New Breasts after Mastectomy 121

Delaying Reconstruction to Complete Breast Cancer Treatment 121
Living with a Flat Chest 123
Saline and Silicone Implants 124
Options for Using Your Own Tissue 127
Optional Last Steps: Adding Nipples and Areolas 131
Great Expectations: Surgery and Recovery 132
Choosing the Right Surgeon 134

CHAPTER 12. Oophorectomy and Other Risk-Reducing Gynecologic Surgeries 138

Oophorectomy Procedures 139
Should You Have a Hysterectomy Too? 143
Oophorectomy, Mastectomy: Either, Neither, or Both? 145
Issues for Breast Cancer Survivors 147

CHAPTER 13. Dealing with Menopause and Quality-of-Life Issues 150

Symptoms of Surgical Menopause 150
Long-Term Side Effects 157
Should You Take Hormones? 160
Issues for Breast Cancer Survivors 163

PART IV. LIVING WITH BRCA: ISSUES AND ANSWERS

CHAPTER 14. Managing Lifestyle Choices 169

The Three-Legged Stool: Nutrition, Weight, and Physical
Activity 170
Alcohol: An Unwise Choice 178
Other Lifestyle Risk Factors 178

CHAPTER 15. Sharing Information with Friends, Family, and Coworkers 183

Sharing Risk and Genetic Testing Information with Family 183
Issues for Spouses, Partners, and People You Date 188
What Should You Tell Employers and Coworkers? 191

CHAPTER 16. Young and at High Risk 194

Should You Consider Testing Now? 194
Diagnostic Difficulties 195
Dealing with a Diagnosis before Menopause 196
Planning Your Family, Preserving Your Fertility 198
Oophorectomy in Young Women 202
Sorting through Emotions 203

CHAPTER 17. How BRCA Affects Men 206

Men Get Breast Cancer Too 207
High Risk for Prostate Cancer 211
Other BRCA-Related Cancers 214

CHAPTER 18. Diagnosis: Hereditary Cancer 217

How Important Is a Second Opinion? 217
Treating Hereditary Cancers 218
Making Breast Cancer Treatment Decisions 220
Ovarian Cancer Issues 222
The Importance of Clinical Trials 224

CHAPTER 19. Putting the Pieces Together to Make Difficult Decisions 228

Start at the Beginning: Should You Be Tested? 228
Making Decisions to Reduce Your Risk 229
Making Decisions about Treatment 233
From Confused to Clear in Fifteen Steps 234

NOTES 237
INDEX 247

Foreword

IT IS BOTH FITTING and instructive that *Confronting Hereditary Breast and Ovarian Cancer* should come to us now, some seventeen years after the identification of the BRCA1 and BRCA2 cancer-susceptibility genes: fitting in that it meets an urgent need for a trusted source of authoritative information, and instructive in demonstrating how far the hereditary breast and ovarian cancer (HBOC) field has progressed since those paradigm-altering observations were made. This important guide can direct our research focus in the years ahead, as we strive to optimize quality of life, management, and survival among persons at increased genetic risk of breast and ovarian cancer.

A glance at the table of contents reveals a comprehensive list of the challenges faced by all carriers of rare cancer-susceptibility genes, ranging from an introduction to genetic principles, through risk assessment and genetic testing, to surgical and medical management, with each topic beautifully illustrated using the specific example of HBOC. The substance of each chapter is impeccably accurate, and the authors honestly acknowledge the limits of our current understanding of this incredibly complex disorder. Where all the facts are not yet known, they present the carefully considered best medical judgment of investigators and providers who have devoted their careers to the study of HBOC, informed and shaped by those carrying BRCA mutations as well as the important people in their lives.

The voices of these women are heard loud and clear throughout the text; they give the information presented here a genuine and legitimate quality that will surely resonate with readers as they struggle to come to terms with what it means to carry a BRCA1/2 mutation. Consequently, the tone of the book is an extraordinary combination of indisputably authoritative and insightful information, presented in a voice that is calm, clear, direct, balanced, realistic, and yet optimistic. Readers will know that, without a doubt, they are hearing from people who have been there and survived, people who now share their hard-won wisdom and insight in an effort to ease the path for those who follow in their footsteps.

The authors employ several novel organizational strategies in an effort to convey their message as clearly as possible. "Expert View" sections give voice to leaders in HBOC research and care; "My Story" sections share the heartfelt words of women who have direct experience with the topic under discussion; and "The FORCE Perspective" sections describe the current positions of the organization that has led the effort to give women from HBOC families a voice in their own fate. All three add greatly to the effectiveness of the educational effort embodied by this book. It is filled with pearls of wisdom that can only come from those who speak from firsthand experience. Examples include the unassailable assertion that genetic counseling must be seen as an ongoing, open-ended process rather than a one-time event, and the discussion of the pros and cons of various surgical approaches to risk-reducing mastectomy.

As a clinician and investigator who has been involved in evaluating HBOC families for the past thirty-five years, since long before the identification of BRCA1/2, I remember all too well the frustrations we faced due to the lack of data upon which to base management recommendations for the pioneering women who participated in our research studies in the 1970s and 1980s. I also remember the anguish of women from multiple-case families who *all* regarded themselves as destined to develop breast and/or ovarian cancer, because of our inability to identify the specific family members who were at genetic risk. It was heartbreaking to realize that many of the women from that era who elected risk-reducing breast and ovarian surgery likely did *not* carry the mutated gene that formed the basis for their family's cancer risk. Perhaps the single greatest difficulty faced by BRCA mutation carriers as they struggled to manage their risk was the lack of reliable, consistent, authoritative information from their healthcare providers, with contradictory recommendations being distressingly common.

This book should go a long way toward making that unacceptable status quo a thing of the past. And for that, future generations of BRCA mutation carriers can thank the indomitable and tireless FORCE organization for insisting that women have the information they need to maximize their long-term survival.

MARK H. GREENE, M.D.
CHIEF, CLINICAL GENETICS BRANCH
NATIONAL CANCER INSTITUTE
BETHESDA, MARYLAND

Acknowledgments

THE AUTHORS gratefully acknowledge the input, support, and enthusiasm of the many people who helped make this book possible. Thank you to all who shared stories and to each and every one of the healthcare professionals and researchers who took the time to contribute an "Expert View."

We appreciate permission to use the filmmaker's statement and a quotation from Kartemquin Films' *In the Family*.

A special thanks to those who read and improved what we wrote, including Diljeet Singh, M.D., Susan Domchek, M.D., Minas Chrysopoulo, M.D., Wendy Rubinstein, M.D., Ph.D., Monica Alvarado, M.S., C.G.C., Jana Pruski-Clark, M.S., C.G.C., Rachel Nussbaum, M.S., C.G.C., Tiffani DeMarco, M.S., Sally Scroggs, R.D., L.D., Jennifer Leib, Sc.M., C.G.C., David Winchester, M.D., Amy Fort, Rose Kovatch, Dan Maysey, Barbara Pfeiffer, and Robin Pugh Yi. Ginger Gardner, M.D., graciously provided timely reviews to help us meet deadlines.

And finally, we are indebted to the extraordinary support of Allison Kurian, M.D., Tim Rebbeck, Ph.D., and Victoria Seewaldt, M.D.

Introduction

THESE DAYS, IT'S NOT UNCOMMON for more than one person in a family to have cancer. Most cancers are not hereditary, but if you or your relatives have been diagnosed, you might wonder how you can learn if the cancers are random or due to some inherited predisposition. Should you be tested to determine whether you've inherited changes in the BReast CAncer1 and BReast CAncer2 (BRCA1 and BRCA2) genes you've heard so much about? Are other risk factors at play? If a test reveals that you have a greater-than-average cancer risk, what should you do to remain cancer free? If you're facing treatment for a diagnosis, how would knowledge of an inherited risk affect you during treatment and beyond?

Sorting through scientific terms, understanding risk management, and dealing with the emotions of it all can be overwhelming. Still, you deserve a "normal" life that isn't disrupted by fears about cancer. If you've inherited high risk or been diagnosed with hereditary breast or ovarian cancer, you face difficult decisions about what is best for you now and in the long term, and you need credible information to make them. You're not the first person to have these concerns or ask these questions. As cancer survivors and women who have pursued genetic counseling and testing, we've asked these same questions ourselves. And as professionals who deal with these medical issues daily, we help people who struggle with the same concerns. We know that confronting hereditary cancer can be a complex, confusing, and highly individual journey. We also know that you can take actions to gain control of your health.

Facing Our Risk of Cancer Empowered (FORCE) was founded on the principle that no one should face hereditary cancer alone. Since 1999, the nonprofit organization has been a trusted source of information, support, and resources for individuals and families affected by hereditary breast and ovarian cancers. For just as long, people have been asking when we would compile that knowledge and expertise into a book. Now we have—you're holding it.

As we put fingers to keyboards, we considered how to develop the most comprehensive and objective resource possible for people wondering what to do about their high cancer risk. We began with our existing base of information, to which we added relevant input from the world's leading cancer and genetics experts. As we wrote about practical risk-reducing alternatives, our goal was to dispel myths and misinformation about hereditary cancer. Then we added a few meaningful extras: personal stories from individuals who have dealt with these same issues and confronted the same agonizing decisions you now face, clarification about insurance coverage and discrimination, unique insights we've learned from serving our community, and a summary of each chapter's key points. The result is *Confronting Hereditary Breast and Ovarian Cancer,* our up-to-date composite of research, insight, and inspiration, all bundled together to provide answers, whether you're new to the subject or well versed.

Decisions about hereditary cancer may be the most difficult you'll ever make. But you needn't make them alone. This book is your road map through the maze of alternatives that comes with living in a high-risk body. We suggest you start at the beginning and read through consecutive chapters. Page by page, you'll sort through and absorb all the information you need, gaining clarity to make the best decisions you can for you and your family. We've organized the book into four main parts:

- "Understanding Cancer, Genetics, and Risk" introduces cancer, specifically breast and ovarian cancer, inherited and acquired genetic damage, and hereditary cancer syndromes that run in families.
- "Assessing Your Risk" explores the value of genetic counseling and genetic testing to determine whether you or someone in your family has a BRCA mutation. This section describes what you can expect from

genetic counseling and testing, which family members should be tested first, how to interpret test results, and how to decipher your range of risk.

- "Managing Your Risk" helps you understand and assess your options for managing and lowering your cancer risk and choose alternatives that are right for you. It also provides decision-making tools and compares different strategies for reducing risk.
- "Living with BRCA" identifies strategies for dealing with the day-to-day and long-term emotional and physical issues of cancer survivors and high-risk individuals. You'll find suggestions for discussing your BRCA status and dealing with the parental guilt of potentially passing along a mutation to your children. You'll read about fertility and family planning issues, sexuality, sensuality, and dating after mastectomy or oophorectomy. Our chapter devoted to men's issues provides information about specific screening, diagnosis, and treatment.

Knowledge can be both empowering and comforting. In many cases, it is lifesaving. And although there is no single right answer for all readers—we are all individuals with our own concerns, circumstances, and priorities that affect our decisions—the information you'll find in this book will demystify the complexities of hereditary cancer.

We can't make decisions for you, but we do the next best thing: we explain all sides of the hereditary cancer story—how to know if you have exceptionally high risk, alternatives for managing that risk, and the benefits and downsides of each choice. You needn't spend hours surfing the Internet looking for information, trying to decipher studies on medical sites, defining terms and attempting to distinguish between hype and fact. We've done that for you. We don't have perfect medical solutions—no one does at this time—but we can help you potentially change your destiny by equipping you with resources, facts, and support.

Be informed. Be empowered. Be well.

SUE FRIEDMAN, D.V.M.
REBECCA SUTPHEN, M.D.
KATHY STELIGO

PART ONE UNDERSTANDING CANCER, GENETICS, AND RISK

Chapter 1 Breast and Ovarian Cancer Basics

FROM A STRICTLY SCIENTIFIC PERSPECTIVE, women have breasts to feed their babies. Yet, for most of us, our breasts are much more than milk-producing glands. Our emotional attachment to our breasts is considerable, increasing as we move from puberty to maturity. Breasts enhance our physical form, give us sexual pleasure, and help us forge a close maternal bond as we nourish our infants. Although our ovaries aren't as visible, their reproductive role is more significant, from our first menstrual cycle to monthly fertility and, finally, our change of life. A woman's breasts and ovaries are uniquely feminine and intensely personal; the threat of cancer in either is particularly scary.

Most Cancers Aren't Hereditary

People with cancer are often surprised if none of their relatives has been diagnosed, but most cancers aren't hereditary. The majority are sporadic. They develop from damage that our genes acquire (not inherit) as we age. Genes are fundamental to all living organisms, including humans. They contain instructions for critical body functions and hold all hereditary information that is passed from parent to child. Inherited genetic changes called *mutations* cause about 5 to 10 percent of breast cancers and 12 percent of ovarian cancers. Most of these hereditary breast and ovarian cancers are caused by mutations in two specific genes, BReast CAncer 1 (BRCA1) and BReast CAncer 2 (BRCA2).[1] These mutations are *familial* (they run in families). They account for only a small percentage of breast and ovarian cancers, yet their presence greatly increases a woman's risk for both. Multiple diagnoses in a family also

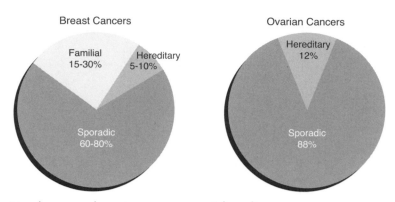

Most breast and ovarian cancers aren't hereditary

raise a woman's risk. A family history of breast cancer, even when there is no BRCA mutation in the family, increases breast cancer risk. A strong history of ovarian cancer elevates a woman's risk for that disease.

Sporadic and hereditary cancers differ in important ways that may affect healthcare decisions:

- Hereditary cancer often occurs at an earlier age than the sporadic form of the same cancer.
- Recommendations for cancer screening and risk reduction can differ, and should begin at a younger age for individuals who have an inherited gene mutation or a family history of cancer.
- Multiple family members may inherit the same gene mutation that increases risk for certain hereditary cancers.
- Children can inherit a parent's gene mutation.

Throughout the remainder of this book, you'll learn how inherited mutations or a family history affect your risk for cancer and how you can manage that risk.

An Introduction to Breast Cancer

More than a million new cases of breast cancer occur each year worldwide. In the United States, it's the second most commonly diagnosed cancer (after skin cancer) among women, and it causes more

Table 1. U.S. breast cancer statistics

Lifetime risk of breast cancer	1 in 8
New cases expected in 2010	261,100*
Estimated deaths in 2010	39,840

Source: American Cancer Society, "What are the risk factors for breast cancer?" www.cancer.org/Cancer/BreastCancer/DetailedGuide/breast-cancer-risk-factors. *Includes 207,090 new cases of invasive breast cancer and 54,010 new cases of noninvasive breast cancer.

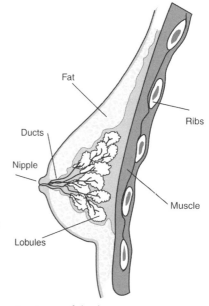

Anatomy of the breast

deaths than any other cancer except lung cancer. It also affects men, although far less frequently—less than 1 percent of all breast cancers occur in men.

Breast cancer deaths have declined since 1990 because of increased awareness, better methods of early detection, and advances in treatment. Yet too many women, about forty thousand every year, still die from this disease. In the 1970s, a woman living in the United States had a 1 in 11 chance of developing breast cancer in her lifetime; those odds steadily worsened over the next two decades. Since 1999, breast cancer has decreased among women over age 50, while rates among younger women remain unchanged. Today, an average woman's lifetime risk of developing breast cancer is 1 in 8 (approximately 12.5 percent) (see table 1).

Breast cancer almost always begins in the lobules (the glands that produce milk) or the ducts (the tubes that carry milk to the nipple). Cancer usually develops over several years, typically without pain or other noticeable symptoms, until it shows up as a suspicious calcification on a mammogram or is found as a lump during a breast exam by a woman or her doctor. A tumor may show itself as it grows: a lump or area of thickness, a change in the size or shape of the breast, a skin irritation or dryness that refuses to heal, or unusual tenderness or discharge from the nipple. These same changes often occur with other conditions and don't always signal breast cancer.

Types of Breast Cancer

Tumors are either in situ, or invasive. In situ, meaning "in place," refers to early stage breast cancer that remains within the ducts or the lobules. Nearly all women diagnosed with in situ breast tumors are cured—their cancer isn't likely to return. Invasive tumors are more worrisome, because if cancerous cells reach the bloodstream or lymph nodes, they can *metastasize* (spread) to the liver, bones, lungs, and other organs. Treatment is then more involved, and remission or cure is less likely.

Ductal carcinoma in situ (DCIS) develops in the milk ducts. About 1 in 5 new breast cancers are DCIS, the earliest stage and most commonly diagnosed in situ breast cancer. Too small to be felt, DCIS is usually found by mammography or magnetic resonance imaging (MRI). Early detection is important because, left untreated, some DCIS develops into invasive breast cancer and may metastasize. If you have DCIS, your risk of developing a new breast cancer or recurrence is higher than that of someone who has never been diagnosed.

Lobular carcinoma in situ (LCIS) isn't considered a true breast cancer. Usually diagnosed in premenopausal women, LCIS involves abnormal cells that signal a higher-than-average risk of developing invasive breast cancer. Rarely found by mammography, LCIS is usually discovered during a breast biopsy to explore a lump, *microcalcification* (the residue from rapidly dividing cells that may signal an early cancer), or other abnormality.

Invasive ductal carcinoma (IDC) is cancer that has spread beyond the ducts to the surrounding breast tissue. It's the most common breast cancer, accounting for about 80 percent of all cases. Although women of any age can develop IDC, it's more often found after age 55.

Invasive lobular carcinoma (ILC) begins in the lobules and spreads to the breast tissue. Only 10 percent of invasive breast cancers are ILC, which is more often diagnosed in women who are age 60 and older.

Inflammatory breast cancer (IBC) accounts for only 1 to 3 percent of breast cancers. It often begins with swelling or reddening of the breast rather than a lump. IBC can grow very quickly—symptoms may worsen in a single day—so it's very important to recognize the signs of this disease and seek prompt treatment. IBC tends to occur at an earlier age than most other breast cancers, on average at age 56 for white women and age 52 for African American women, who are more likely to develop IBC.

Paget's disease spreads from the ducts to the nipple or areola and is often characterized by a dry, scaly, itchy, or red patch. It usually affects women 50 and older. Paget's is quite rare, less than 1 percent of all breast cancers. Because most women with Paget's disease also have DCIS or invasive breast cancer, early diagnosis is very important.

> **STAGING CANCERS**
>
> By defining a tumor's size, how far it has spread, and whether lymph nodes are involved, *oncologists* (cancer experts) *stage* cancers to develop a treatment plan and predict a patient's long-term outcome. Stage 0 is sometimes called pre-invasive cancer and includes DCIS. Stages 1 to 3 depend on tumor size and lymph node involvement. Stage 4 cancers have metastasized and invaded other organs.

Tumor Characteristics

Cancers have different characteristics, and no two are exactly alike. Some are slow growing and predictable. Others grow aggressively. A tumor's size, stage, and growth pattern determine how it's treated. Some breast cancers have hormone receptors: protein molecules in the cells that bind to estrogen and progesterone and act like on-off switches for tumor growth. Cancers with hormone receptors are referred to as *estrogen receptor–positive* (ER+) or *progesterone receptor–positive* (PR+); they respond well to antihormone treatments that either reduce the amount of estrogen or progesterone in the body or block a tumor's ability to use these hormones to grow. ER+ and PR+ tumors usually occur in women who are older than age 50. They're also the most common tumors in women with BRCA2 mutations, regardless of age. Tumors without estrogen or progesterone receptors are said to be receptor-negative (ER– and PR–); they don't respond as well to antihormone therapies. Up to a third of breast cancers *overexpress* (make too much) *HER2/neu*, a protein that promotes the growth of cancer cells. Treatment includes medications that specifically target HER2 receptors.

About 15 percent of breast cancers are *triple-negative*; they're not sensitive to estrogen, progesterone, or HER2. These cancers occur more often before age 50, especially in women who are African American or who have a BRCA1 mutation. Triple-negative tumors don't respond to hormone therapies or treatments that target the HER2 protein. Research of potential new drugs to treat triple-negative breast cancers is promising.

An Introduction to Ovarian Cancer

Ovaries are two small glands that are part of the female reproductive system, along with the fallopian tubes, vagina, and uterus. During puberty, a girl's ovaries begin to produce estrogen, progesterone, and testosterone as she develops into a sexually mature woman, and

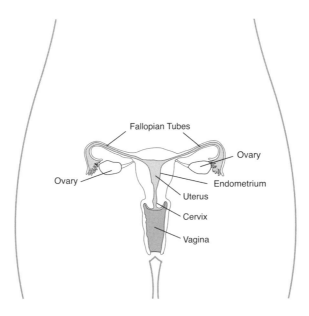

Female reproductive system

her body prepares for childbearing. During monthly ovulation, one ovary releases an egg, which then travels through the fallopian tube to the uterus. If the egg is fertilized with sperm, conception occurs. If it remains unfertilized, it dries up and is shed during menstruation.

Our ovaries produce estrogen, progesterone, and other hormones that control fertility, support pregnancy, and affect other critical body functions during our reproductive years. Ovaries keep bones strong, boost metabolism, stimulate sex drive, and regulate the menstrual cycle. As you age and reach menopause, your ovaries gradually produce fewer hormones, until your menstrual periods stop.

We don't know exactly why cancer develops in the ovaries. Some experts theorize that the monthly process of releasing eggs may cause damage that eventually leads to cancer. Others believe that the balance of progesterone compared to estrogen may play a role in protecting the ovaries from cancer. The risk for ovarian cancer increases as we age, and most ovarian cancers develop after menopause. Half develop in women over age 63.

Ovarian cancer isn't as common as breast cancer, but the ovaries are tucked away deep in the body, and without reliable early detection, tumors aren't usually discovered until they've progressed to an advanced stage and are more difficult to treat. Most early stage breast and ovarian cancers are cured, yet only about 20 percent of ovarian cancers are discovered at an early stage before they've spread to other tissue or organs. Although women diagnosed in the earliest stages have a five-year survival rate of nearly 93 percent—nearly double what it was twenty years ago—the number of ovarian cancer cases found early remains small (see table 2).

Table 2. U.S. ovarian cancer statistics

Lifetime risk of invasive ovarian cancer	1 in 70
New cases expected in 2010	21,880
Estimated deaths in 2010	13,850

Source: American Cancer Society, "What are the key statistics about ovarian cancer?" www.cancer.org/Cancer/OvarianCancer/DetailedGuide/ovarian-cancer-key-statistics.

Ovarian Cancer Symptoms

Ovarian cancer has been termed "the silent killer" because it was falsely believed to be a disease without warning signs. But research confirms that many women experience symptoms several months before they're diagnosed. Being aware of symptoms could lead to earlier diagnosis. Symptoms can include:

- bloating
- pelvic or abdominal pain
- difficulty eating or feeling full quickly
- change in urinary urgency or frequency
- fatigue
- indigestion
- back pain
- pain during intercourse
- constipation
- menstrual irregularities

These symptoms can be subtle and easily ignored or mistakenly associated with bladder or digestive conditions. Symptoms are particularly significant if they're new, occur every other day or more frequently, and last more than two weeks. If your doctor treats you for something other than ovarian cancer, and your symptoms linger or become worse, quickly get a second opinion from a gynecologic expert. Surviving ovarian cancer depends on early detection.

Ovarian and Related Cancers

About 90 percent of ovarian cancers (and most hereditary ovarian cancers) are believed to begin in the epithelial cells that form a thin layer of tissue covering the ovary. When experts refer to ovarian cancer risk, symptoms, and diagnosis, they're including *primary peritoneal* and *fallopian tube* cancers, which are treated similarly to ovarian cancer.

Fallopian tube cancer. Fallopian tube cancer affects only three hundred to four hundred women in the United States annually, usually between ages 50 and 60. Symptoms may include abdominal pain or pressure and unusual vaginal bleeding (especially after menopause) or discharge. Emerging research suggests that many hereditary ovarian cancers may actually be fallopian tube cancers that have spread to the ovaries; distinguishing between the two can be challenging. The lifetime risk for BRCA-related fallopian tube cancer is relatively low, about 6 percent.[2]

Primary peritoneal cancer. Primary peritoneal cancer begins outside the ovaries in the peritoneum, a thin membrane lining the abdomen, and can very quickly spread to other tissues. The peritoneum is made up of the same type of epithelial cells that line the ovaries, so it's not surprising that peritoneal cancer looks and behaves like ovarian cancer, has similar symptoms, and is treated as stage 3 or 4 ovarian cancer. Women with high risk for ovarian cancer, particularly those with inherited risk, are more likely to also develop peritoneal cancer, although it occurs rarely. The lifetime risk for BRCA-related primary peritoneal cancer is 2 to 6 percent.[3]

Other Hereditary Cancers

Families with BRCA1 or BRCA2 mutations have increased risk for breast and ovarian cancer. They may also have higher-than-average risk for other cancers. (Screening recommendations for these cancers are discussed in chapter 8. Other cancers caused by mutations in different genes, which can run in families, are discussed in chapter 4.)

Pancreatic Cancer

The pancreas aids digestion, secretes insulin, and regulates your body's sugar level. Because the pancreas is positioned behind the stomach, tumors are difficult to detect. Even when it's diagnosed early, this disease spreads quickly and is difficult to treat. Risk factors include:

- aging, especially after age 60
- being overweight or obese
- smoking
- diabetes
- being African American
- a family history of certain hereditary cancers
- a personal or family history of pancreatic cancer

Pancreatic cancer is uncommon; the average person's lifetime risk is just 1 percent. Family history is an important predictor. Having two first-degree relatives with this disease raises risk by a factor of 18; three or more relatives with the disease equates to a 57-fold increase in risk.[4] BRCA mutation carriers have increased lifetime risk that is still quite small: 2 percent with a BRCA1 mutation and 3 to 5 percent with a BRCA2 mutation.[5] Inherited mutations are linked to about 10 percent of pancreatic cancers, even when there's no family history of the disease. If pancreatic cancer runs in your family, consult with a genetics specialist to determine your risk and to develop a plan for risk management.

> **PREVIVOR OR SURVIVOR?**
>
> If you've ever been diagnosed with cancer, you're a *survivor*. You're a *previvor* if you have a family history of disease, an inherited mutation, or other factor that predisposes you to developing cancer and you've never been diagnosed.

Melanoma

People with mutations in BRCA2 have a slightly increased risk for melanoma, an aggressive and deadly form of cancer that affects the skin and eyes. Excessive exposure to sunlight is a risk factor for both cancers, especially if you have naturally blonde or red hair, fair skin, and blue or green eyes. Melanoma of the eye often presents no symptoms, especially in its early stages. It may cause blurred vision in one eye, floaters (small spots that move around in your field of vision), a spot or a change of color on the iris, pain in the eye, or loss of peripheral vision. The lifetime risk for BRCA2-related melanoma is about 5 percent.[6]

Prostate Cancer

Men with BRCA mutations have increased risk for prostate cancer (discussed in chapter 17).

WHAT TO REMEMBER ABOUT BREAST AND OVARIAN CANCER

- Breast cancer may develop with no noticeable symptoms.
- Many women who develop ovarian cancer do have symptoms.
- Breast cancer is often discovered in its early, most treatable stages. Ovarian cancer is not.
- Most cancers aren't caused by an inherited mutation.

LEARN MORE ABOUT BREAST AND OVARIAN CANCER

The American Cancer Society (www.cancer.org) offers information and support related to prevention, treatment, and research involving all types of cancers.

Susan G. Komen for the Cure (www.cancer.org) and www.breastcancer .org provide up-to-date information about breast cancer.

The National Ovarian Cancer Coalition (www.ovarian.org) and the Ovarian Cancer National Alliance (www.ovariancancer.org) provide support and information related to ovarian cancer.

Chapter 2   **A Peek Inside**

Your Genes at Work

FEW AREAS OF SCIENCE HAVE CHANGED THE WORLD of medicine more in the past fifty years than genetics, the study of hereditary characteristics and variations passed from parent to child. With capabilities previously unimagined, scientists use genetic processes to trace ancestry, examine fossils, and make foods more disease resistant. Because most diseases, including breast and ovarian cancers, are caused at least in part by changes in the genes, this science is the key to understanding the origins of disease. Blood tests can now detect genetic changes that can cause diseases, from cystic fibrosis in a newborn to breast and ovarian cancer in an adult. Knowing about these genetic disorders can be life changing, because it provides opportunities to reduce the likelihood of developing the disease or to manage it early on. These discoveries are amazing, yet they only scratch the genetic surface. The more scientists understand what causes genetic abnormalities that lead to cancer, the closer we move toward better prevention, detection, treatment, and cure.

The Evolution of Genetic Discovery: From Peas to BRCA

In 1866, Austrian monk Gregor Mendel, considered the father of genetics, made a stunning declaration based on his experiments crossbreeding pea plants: that "factors" (now called genes) determine traits that are passed unchanged to descendants, and for each trait, individuals inherit one gene from each parent. Science ultimately proved Mendel correct and his conclusions became the tenets of modern genetics. Genes pass from parent to child, along with abnormalities within the genes that raise a person's risk for disease.

In 1990, genetics researcher Dr. Mary-Claire King demonstrated that a single inherited gene mutation causes breast and ovarian cancer among multiple members in some families. The link between the two cancers had been suspected since the late 1800s; now researchers had a clue for further exploration. Her proof that breast cancers could be inherited paved the way for subsequent research. King documented the general location of the "breast cancer" gene. A frenzy of subsquent research followed, and in 1994, scientists documented the precise location of BRCA1, the first breast cancer gene, on chromosome 17. BRCA2 was identified on chromosome 13 the following year. Now researchers knew exactly where to find these two genes, and a blood test was developed to screen individuals for cancer-causing BRCA mutations.

In the same year Dr. King announced her discovery, the Human Genome Project was launched to identify the entire set of human genes. By 2003, researchers had successfully labeled all 20,000 or so genes and created a genetic road map showing where each could be found. The massive effort was akin to translating every book ever written into a universal language: the genetic code that enables researchers to study what each gene does and how abnormalities cause disease. Even though it will be several years before we have all the answers, the increasing pace of genetic discoveries is rapidly advancing our knowledge of disease. Because genes appear in exactly the same order in all of us, knowing the location of a particular disease-causing gene is a huge medical leap forward. We now know where to find more than four thousand genes related to diseases, including many cancers.

Discovering BRCA1/2 was an important step in identifying high-risk individuals and finding ways to reduce their breast and ovarian cancer risk. As we learn more about BRCA mutations, our arsenal of risk management tools and cancer treatments grows. We still have much to learn about hereditary cancer. We don't know why some people with mutations get breast cancer and others develop ovarian cancer, or why some never have either disease. We can't predict when cancer will develop or how individuals will respond to treatment. And there may be as-yet undiscovered gene mutations that also raise cancer risk. Future genetic discoveries will provide those answers, ultimately leading to methods that will eradicate these diseases.

Your Genetic ABCs . . . and a D

Genetics is a complex science with its own unique language. Understanding the basics helps to clarify how changes in BRCA genes can lead to increased cancer risk.

A is for All of Us

Geraniums, worms, poodles, and humans—all living organisms have the same fundamental microscopic cells that keep us operating. Humans have trillions of cells, each with the same basic structure, yet programmed for very specific tasks like breathing, converting food into energy, and sending messages to and from the brain. You have an almost unimaginable assortment of cells, and most of them contain a complete set of your genetic material sufficient to create an exact copy of you.

B is for the Basics

Within each of our cells (except red blood cells) is a genetic control center called the nucleus. Every nucleus has twenty-three pairs of chromosomes: one of each pair comes from your mother; the other is from your father. Chromosomes are composed of snippets of genetic material that store and transmit the operating instructions that keep our bodies functioning. Genes also come in pairs (except those in egg and sperm cells), one from each parent. Genes work together to determine specific human characteristics, such as height or hair color, that pass from one generation to the next. When someone says, "It's in your genes," they're referring to a characteristic that's very much like one of your parent's. They might mean the curly hair both you and your mother have or the artistic ability you share with your father. Some genetic characteristics, such as eye color or the shape of your hairline, don't affect your health or well-being. Others may cause traits like color blindness or make you more likely to develop diseases such as diabetes or breast cancer.

C is for Cells

We all begin life as a single cell that grows and divides. Those two cells then divide and become four, and so on and so on, until our bodies are formed. This replicating life cycle is normally carried out in an orderly process controlled by genes: some tell cells when to divide, and others put the brakes on cell growth.

D is for DNA

You've probably heard of DNA, which stands for *deoxyribonucleic acid,* the unique genetic material used to link suspects to crime scenes, prove someone's paternity, or screen for certain mutations that lead to disease. All humans share about 99.9 percent of our DNA. Yet, except for identical twins, no two people are exactly alike. That's because our individual one-tenth of a percent variation determines our inherited

A genetic portrait of your DNA

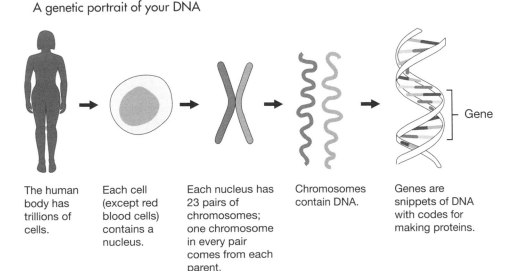

The human body has trillions of cells.

Each cell (except red blood cells) contains a nucleus.

Each nucleus has 23 pairs of chromosomes; one chromosome in every pair comes from each parent.

Chromosomes contain DNA.

Genes are snippets of DNA with codes for making proteins.

Gene

traits, like eye color and hair texture. Although you and your sister have genes that determine eye color, your variation of those genes may have resulted in your eyes being brown, while your sister's unique genetic variation gave her hazel eyes.

Genes perform an incredibly important job. These tightly coiled sections of thin DNA fibers issue instructions for making the thousands of proteins that build and support the body's elaborate operations—move muscles, digest food, repair cell damage. We hear a lot these days about genes, but proteins—often referred to as the body's building blocks—are the chemicals of life, and every cellular function depends on them. Genes instruct cells which proteins to make based on the type of cell and its needs. Some, like BRCA genes, tell our bodies how to repair damage from sun exposure, chemicals, and other influences. Others maintain just the right number of cells—enough to keep the body healthy, but not too many to encourage tumor growth. Cells, chromosomes, DNA, genes, proteins—mix these elements together uniquely and the result is: you.

Mutations: Spelling Errors in Your DNA Cookbook

Think of DNA as your body's cookbook, where your genes are recipes for proteins made by your body. DNA recipes are written in a sort of biological shorthand using various combinations of a four-letter alphabet, each representing a different chemical base: A (adenine), C (cytosine), G (guanine), and T (thymine). By combining different variations of these four "letters" into three-letter "words," DNA issues instructions for all the proteins our bodies need. The unique order of these letters spells out recipes for making everything from

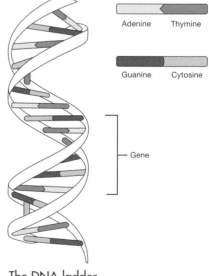

Adenine   Thymine

Guanine   Cytosine

Gene

The DNA ladder

Table 3. Genetic spelling errors

Intended recipe	Mutation (spelling error)	Result
Add one big egg	Delete one letter (recipe begins in the wrong place and words shift)	Ddo neb ige gg
	Insert one letter (recipe shifts)	Add don ebi geg g
	Substitute letters	Add one bug egg
	Rearrangements	Egg add one big

hormones to heart valves. Under the microscope, DNA molecules look like the rungs of a ladder made up of A-T and C-G pairs.

If you use a cake recipe that includes a typo, your dessert might not turn out the way it should. The same thing happens when genetic changes called mutations create "spelling errors" that garble a DNA recipe for a specific protein. Different types of spelling errors may occur (see table 3).

Some spelling errors completely change the recipe and make it unreadable. Insertions and deletions cause words to shift, resulting in nonsense. Substitution errors can create sentences made up of real words that have different meanings: adding a "bug" egg instead of a "big" egg ruins the recipe. Sometimes, even though all the right letters are there, they end up in the wrong place, or words become scrambled and create meaningless sentences, creating mutations called *rearrangements*.

Most mutations aren't harmful. Some play an important evolutionary role, like changing an animal's appearance or behavior in ways that better adapt it to its surroundings. In some cases, the end result of mutations is disease. Sickle cell anemia, for instance, occurs when a mutation disrupts the instructions for hemoglobin, a protein made by red blood cells to move oxygen through the bloodstream. Mutations can also develop naturally as we grow older, as the wear and tear of living takes its toll on our recuperative abilities, and our genetic repair mechanisms don't work as effectively as they used to. Cells often develop mutations when they divide, and other mutations occur as a result of environmental and

MUTATIONS ARE ACQUIRED OR INHERITED

Like property and wealth, genetic mutations can be acquired or inherited. You might earn $50,000 or inherit the same amount. Similarly, you can accumulate or inherit mutations. Acquired mutations are limited to cells where the damage occurs. Too much sun exposure can impair your skin cells and cause an age spot, for example. When the damaged skin cells divide, the new cells they create will have the same genetic damage and produce the same age spot—that's acquired damage. That damage, however, doesn't extend to all the other cells in your body or to egg or sperm cells, so your children won't inherit your corrupted skin cells (although they might acquire age spots of their own). Inherited mutations, on the other hand, exist in all cells, including egg or sperm cells, and can be passed from you to your children.

lifestyle influences, such as chemical exposure, radiation, smoking, and alcohol. The body frequently repairs genetic damage before the mutation is copied to new cells. Damage that cannot be repaired creates a bit of a vicious cycle: when a damaged cell divides, it passes all its DNA code, including any unrepaired mutations, on to the next generation of new cells. That error is then copied every time the new cell duplicates itself. If an error occurs in the egg or sperm, it may pass from parent to child in successive generations.

How Mutations Lead to Cancer

Not all cells divide—brain and heart cells don't. Those that do are more likely to develop mutations. Experts believe that cancer develops when both copies of certain genes in one cell are damaged and can't be repaired. Healthy cells usually repair DNA damage. Having two copies of each damage-repairing gene acts as a backup repair system: if one gene can't repair damage, the other can. That's why being born with a single BRCA mutation doesn't guarantee you'll develop breast or ovarian cancer, because your remaining BRCA gene can repair damage. If you develop a single error in that remaining protective BRCA gene, the damage control process is deactivated, and the gene no longer makes proteins to repair damage within the cells. When that first cell divides, it creates more damaged, unregulated copies of

How cell mutations evolve into cancer

 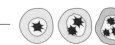 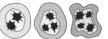 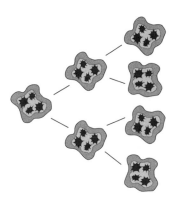

Normal cell   Cell mutations   Uncontrolled growth

itself. These cells are then free to run amok, growing and dividing beyond their normal lifespan and forming a tumor. On average, a breast tumor develops over six to eight years before it's large enough to be found by a mammogram, and about ten years before it can be felt. The process may occur sooner in people with hereditary mutations because the first step in cancer development—disabling one copy of the protective gene—has already occurred.

**GENE THERAPY:
A GLIMPSE INTO THE FUTURE**

When cars malfunction or limbs break, we fix them. Can we do the same with rogue genes? Scientists are studying ways to repair faulty genes or override their cancer-causing ways. Someday, mutated BRCA genes might be fixed or swapped for healthy replacements.

EXPERT VIEW: Gene Variations and Breast Cancer Risk

BY KENNETH OFFIT, M.D., M.P.H.

Two categories of genes are associated with increased breast cancer risk. The first are genes in which mutations are quite rare, including BRCA1 and BRCA2, TP53, PTEN, STK11, and others, which are associated with greatly increased risk. A subset of this group includes ATM, CHEK2, BRIP1, PALB2, and other genes with rare mutations that are linked to much higher risks than those in the general population yet lower than with BRCA.

The second group includes a number of *single-nucleotide polymorphisms* (SNPs), genetic variations that only slightly increase breast cancer risk.

(continued)

Although SNPs occur in 10 to 30 percent or more of the population, the risk for breast cancer they cause is small: a 1.1- to 1.3-fold increased risk for individual SNPs compared to the 20- to 50-fold increased risk for breast cancer from BRCA mutations. Adding these new genetic variants to traditional risk models such as the Gail Model (see chapter 3) provides little new information that is clinically useful.

For now, SNPs are still poorly understood by scientists and best used in research. Although commercial laboratories market breast cancer SNP tests to the public, the American Society of Clinical Oncology and other professional groups caution about the potential harms of using unproven tests to determine risk. Several research groups are exploring whether SNPs can explain multiple cases of breast cancer in families who have no mutations in known breast cancer genes.

BRCA1 and BRCA2 testing continues to represent only the tip of the iceberg in pinpointing the link between genes and cancer risk, yet it remains the most reliable means to assess hereditary risk. In the future, we can expect more extensive evaluation of an individual's complete genetic information and a better understanding of how variations among genes can predispose us to disease. This will provide people with estimates of their risk for cancer and other diseases, as well as their sensitivities to certain environmental exposures and to drugs that may be prescribed to prevent breast and other cancers.

What's So Special about BRCA?

Hereditary breast and ovarian cancer doesn't develop because we have BRCA genes; everyone has them. It's mutations in these genes that cause disease. BRCA1 and BRCA2 are important because they're *tumor-suppressor* genes—their normal role is to stop cancer from developing by helping cells repair DNA damage. Most hereditary breast and ovarian cancers are caused by mutations in these genes. Mutations in other tumor-suppressor genes may also cause cancer.

Although BRCA mutations are found in all races and ethnicities, they're most prevalent in people of Ashkenazi Jewish descent. One in 40 will test positive, compared to 1 in 350 to 500 in the general population.[1] At some point far back in history, Ashkenazi ancestors developed DNA defects in some of their genes, including in BRCA1 and BRCA2. These *founder* mutations have been passed from generation to generation with greater frequency than in other populations because the Ashkenazi have lived in relative isolation, maintaining their common gene pool. About 40 percent of Jewish women with ovarian cancer and 20 percent who have premenopausal breast cancer have a BRCA mutation—a much higher rate than non-Jewish populations. Some Hispanic people (mostly those of Mexican heritage) carry the same mutation commonly found in Ashkenazi Jews, possibly due to a shared Spanish ancestry.[2] BRCA mutations also occur more often among Icelanders, Norwegians, Dutch, French Canadians, and other ethnic groups with relatively small numbers of ancestors.

You're more likely to have a BRCA mutation if your family has any of the following features:

- Ashkenazi Jewish heritage
- Any family member with
    - ovarian, fallopian tube, or primary peritoneal cancer at any age
    - breast cancer at age 50 or younger
    - breast cancer in both breasts at any age
    - both breast and ovarian cancer
    - male breast cancer
- More than one relative on the same side of the family with
    - breast cancer
    - ovarian, fallopian tube, or primary peritoneal cancer
    - prostate cancer
    - pancreatic cancer

WHAT TO REMEMBER ABOUT GENETICS

- All humans have exactly the same number of genes.
- Genetic mutations can be acquired or inherited.
- Mutations can interfere with a gene's ability to repair cellular damage.
- Cancer occurs when cells grow uncontrollably.

LEARN MORE ABOUT GENETICS

Genetics Home Reference (ghr.nlm.nih.gov) is a comprehensive guide for understanding genetics, including an A-to-Z guide to genetic conditions.

A Revolution in Progress: Human Genetics and Medical Research (history.nih.gov/exhibits/genetics/index.htm) is an illustrated introduction to the genetic influence on disease.

Breakthrough: The Race to Find the Breast Cancer Gene, by Kevin Davies and Michael White, describes the historic efforts to identify the BRCA1 gene.

Chapter 3 Defining Risk

DO YOU WORRY about getting malaria? Probably not if you live in the United States, where our risk of that disease is slim. But like many women, you may fear your risk of cancer, especially when you hear that 1 in 8 women will develop breast cancer. This means that, based on current rates of breast cancer in the entire U.S. population of women, 1 of 8 women born now will develop the disease by age 85. That sounds like a lot, but it also means that 7 of 8 women won't be diagnosed. Ovarian cancer occurs less often; the average woman has just a 1 in 70 chance in her lifetime.

The 1 in 8 and 1 in 70 estimates represent the average woman's risk for breast and ovarian cancer, yet these are broad statistics that don't define what you need to know to address your own risk: what is it now and how will it change as you grow older? If you're 20 years old now with an average risk for breast cancer, you have a 1 in 8 chance of being diagnosed in your lifetime. Your current risk isn't 1 in 8. It's much lower and gradually increases as you age (most risk occurs after

U.S. lifetime breast and ovarian cancer rates

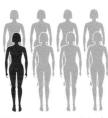

Breast cancer: 1 in 8

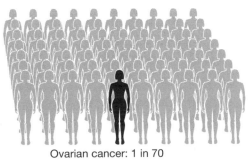

Ovarian cancer: 1 in 70

age 50). Until we know all the causes of cancer, we can't be sure about an individual's exact risk. In the meantime, scientists use population-based figures to describe the frequency of a disease, to help public health officials develop screening guidelines, and to determine cancer trends.

Making Sense of Statistics

Breast cancer is one of the most studied diseases in the world, yet most women don't know much about their own risk. Even fewer understand their odds of developing ovarian cancer. The concept of cancer risk can be confusing—just hearing *risk* is chilling—and because it's often expressed in different ways, understanding how it applies to you can be difficult.

Certain factors raise your likelihood of disease: having high blood pressure increases your chance of developing heart disease, obesity boosts the odds of diabetes, and inheriting a BRCA mutation significantly raises your probability for breast and ovarian cancer. There are many reasons why your chance of developing cancer differs from someone else's, and therein lies the complexity, if not the impossibility, of pinpointing a person's exact risk. Your own risk of breast cancer isn't 1 in 8 because you're not average. It's a moving target that changes throughout your lifetime, depending on your family history, age, race and ethnicity, lifestyle, and other factors that shift your odds of developing cancer higher or lower than the population average. Although risk assessment is never an exact science, it's becoming more precise as researchers continue to learn about factors that influence cancer. Fortunately, genetics experts can assess different aspects of your personal medical history and family history to help you better predict and understand your risk. Confronting that risk may be

> **CALCULATING THE 1 IN 8 STATISTIC**
>
> The current 1 in 8 statistic is calculated by the National Cancer Institute based on breast cancer rates in the United States between 2001 and 2003, when 12.5 percent of women were diagnosed. That statistic will change as breast cancer rates increase or decrease.

frightening, but it's critical to do so, especially if you're genetically predisposed to one or more cancers, because if your risk is high, you have options for managing it.

EXPERT VIEW: Risk Assessment Using the Gail Model

BY VICTORIA SEEWALDT, M.D.

Experts use several tools, including the popular Gail Model, to estimate a woman's breast cancer risk. This model considers a woman's most common risk factors compared to women in the general population, based on her age; her age at first childbirth and menstrual period; whether her mother, sister, or daughter had breast cancer; and the number of breast biopsies she's had. It isn't the best way to determine hereditary breast cancer risk for several reasons:

- The model takes into account only first-degree female relatives, ignoring all other relatives including paternal history.
- It doesn't consider other cancers that can increase risk, such as ovarian cancer in a female relative or male breast cancer.
- It doesn't take into account the age when breast cancer occurs.
- It underestimates breast cancer risk in women of color.

MY STORY: The Gail Model Didn't Work for Me

My mother was diagnosed at age 31 and died four years later. My grandmother and great-grandmother also had breast cancer, and I wondered if there was a hereditary link. I asked my primary care physician about genetic testing, reminding him that my mother had been diagnosed at my age. He told me his nurse had just received a risk tool called the Gail Model that could assess my risk. Based on my answers to just seven questions, she determined I wasn't at high risk. I was relieved, but I couldn't stop thinking about one of the questions she had asked repeatedly: "How many of your sisters or your mother's sisters developed breast cancer?" My answer had been zero, because neither of us had any sisters. Would a different answer affect my risk assessment? I realized the test didn't apply to me because I

(continued)

had few female relatives. I needed someone more qualified, and that led me to genetic counseling and then genetic testing, which showed I have a BRCA1 mutation and my risk is actually quite high.   —JORDAN

Getting Personal: Factors That Modify Your Risk

Risk is the probability of something occurring at a certain time. When you drive to work each day, you take the chance of getting stuck in traffic or being rear-ended. Climb a ladder and you risk falling off. We're all susceptible to the risk of developing certain cancers, even though our risk is not the same. Having one or more risk factors—including a BRCA mutation—doesn't guarantee you'll develop cancer. It means you're more likely to do so. Smoking, for example, increases the odds of developing lung cancer. Stop smoking, and you decrease that risk. Obesity is a contributing risk factor for some diseases; maintaining a healthy weight has the opposite effect. You can control numerous lifestyle factors to reduce your risk; others you cannot. The following factors affect breast and ovarian cancer risk in the general population and, in some cases, may also influence risk in women with BRCA mutations.

Breast and ovarian cancer risk factors you cannot control:

- Being female. All women are at risk for breast and ovarian cancer.
- Growing older. Your risk increases as you age, whether or not you have a BRCA mutation.
- Personal history of breast cancer. Surviving breast cancer increases your risk for another diagnosis whether or not you have a BRCA mutation. The risk is greater for women with mutations.
- Inheriting a genetic mutation. Having a BRCA mutation raises the risk for breast and ovarian cancer more than any other factor. Other inherited mutations may also raise cancer risk (discussed in chapter 4).
- A family history of breast or ovarian cancer. Having a family history of cancer influences risk, although it's difficult to predict how much. About 1 in 4 women with breast cancer has a relative who has also been diagnosed; most don't have a BRCA mutation. If your family has

multiple members with breast cancer, no history of ovarian cancer, and no known BRCA mutation, your estimated lifetime risk for breast cancer is 20 to 25 percent.[1] Your lifetime risk for ovarian cancer is 1.4 percent (the same as an average woman's).[2] Having relatives diagnosed with ovarian cancer raises your risk for a similar diagnosis, even when you have no known mutation. Within BRCA families, having more cancers among relatives appears to cause higher breast and ovarian cancer risk for women family members. No matter what your family history, a genetics expert can help explain your personal risk.

- Race and ethnicity. Certain populations are more likely to develop breast cancer. Compared to white women, African American women have lower rates of breast and ovarian cancer but are more likely to be diagnosed before age 40. Their breast tumors are often particularly aggressive or triple-negative cancers that don't respond to hormone-blocking therapy, and their breast cancer mortality rate is higher than any other group of U.S. women.[3] Hispanic women are also diagnosed less frequently than their white counterparts. When they develop breast cancer, their tumors are more likely to be advanced. Among Asian women, breast cancer occurs less frequently, but it's increasing at a faster rate.

- Very high radiation exposure. Receiving radiation to your chest as a child or young adult elevates your risk of developing breast cancer later in life.

- Age at first menstruation. Early menarche increases the risk for breast cancer in the general population and may have the same effect in women with BRCA mutations.

- Previous breast biopsies. Having any number of biopsies, especially if they showed certain precancerous breast changes, can indicate increased breast cancer risk.

- Breast density. Women with dense breast tissue have greater risk of developing breast cancer, LCIS, and other precancerous abnormalities.

- Infertility. Though research is limited and the connection is unclear, infertility has been linked to increased breast cancer risk in BRCA carriers and to breast and ovarian cancer risk in the general population.

Breast and ovarian cancer risk factors you can modify:

You can't totally eliminate your risk for cancer, but you can change your behavior to reduce your risk. The following factors affect breast and ovarian cancer risk to different degrees in the general population and, in some cases, also influence risk in BRCA carriers. In subsequent chapters, you'll read more about how you can modify these lifestyle factors to change your risk.

- Pregnancy. Being pregnant affects breast cancer risk in complex ways. For all women, a first pregnancy while young lowers risk—the younger you are, the more beneficial the effect. If you're a previvor, your risk may also be affected by your number of pregnancies and whether you have a mutation in BRCA1 or BRCA2.
- Oral contraceptives. Using oral contraceptives while young and continuing for more than five years may increase breast cancer risk in women with BRCA mutations (research is limited). On the other hand, oral contraceptives lower the chance for ovarian cancer in all women.
- Tubal ligation. In the general population, tying a woman's tubes may lower her risk for ovarian cancer, although not as much as oral contraceptives do. Whether this is true for high-risk women is unknown.
- Hormone replacement therapy. Women of average breast cancer risk who take combined estrogen and progesterone hormone replacement after natural menopause have increased risk for breast and ovarian cancer. Hormones may be safer for previvors who pre-emptively remove their breasts and ovaries than for women in the general population, who have undergone natural menopause.
- Alcohol consumption. Having one or more drinks a day elevates the chance of breast cancer in women of average risk. Researchers aren't sure whether women with BRCA mutations are affected in the same way.
- Exercise and obesity. Evidence suggests that physical activity and maintaining an ideal body weight (avoiding obesity) lower the odds of developing breast cancer in women of average or high risk.
- Breast reduction. Some preliminary (and not widely validated) research indicates that breast cancer risk is reduced after breast reduction surgery.

- Removing both breasts and ovaries. These aggressive preventive actions reduce your risk.

It's a Numbers Game

Calculating someone's precise risk for BRCA-related breast and ovarian cancer is difficult. It's a field that is still evolving, and we simply don't know everything about it, including other genes or factors that might also influence risk. BRCA risk estimates are calculated from studies of large multicancer families, and it's unclear how much risk is due to genetic mutations or environmental influences shared by family members. In the absence of finite predictions, genetics experts use a range of numbers to describe a person's odds of developing cancer; even this range of risk varies. Experts may not agree on the exact numbers, but they do agree that inheriting a BRCA mutation means higher-than-average risk that warrants increased surveillance or risk-reducing strategies.

Absolute and Relative Risk

It's important to understand two distinctly different types of risk. *Absolute risk* is the chance of getting cancer over a certain period. The 1 in 8 breast cancer statistic, for example, expresses an average woman's lifetime risk if she lives to age 85. Absolute risk is never less than 0 or more than 100 percent. *Relative risk* is

YOUR BELIEFS AND CULTURE MAY AFFECT HOW YOU CONFRONT YOUR RISK

We all have different ideas about medicine and cancer risk that are often shaped by how we were raised, our family beliefs, and our observations of others who have been diagnosed. Concerns about modesty may prevent you from learning more about cancers of your breasts and ovaries or even speaking about these issues. Social and economic influences may keep you from performing self-exams, having routine mammograms, or changing lifestyle behaviors that affect your risk. Some cultures consider illness to be a *fait accompli;* it's accepted as a destiny we can't control, so why worry about it or try to prevent it? Perhaps you're mistrustful or disillusioned because you can't find a physician who speaks your preferred language. You may feel stigmatized by a cancer diagnosis and delay recommended treatment. Culture and shared values connect us to family and community, which provide our support system, but sometimes it's wise to take a step back and assess if our beliefs help or hinder how we approach important health issues.

Lifetime breast and ovarian cancer risk as a percentage

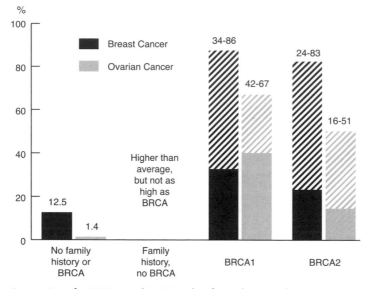

Source: Data for BRCA1 and BRCA2 taken from Chen S and Parmigiani G, "Meta-Analysis of BRCA1 and BRCA2 Penetrance," *Journal of Clinical Oncology* 25, no. 11 (2007): 1329–33.

a percentage of increase or decrease calculated by comparing people who have a particular risk factor with people who don't; in other words, a smoker compared to a nonsmoker. Consider an average woman whose lifetime risk for breast cancer is 12.5 percent. Something that inflates her relative risk by 10 percent raises her absolute risk to 13.75 percent (12.5 + 1.25). If a woman with a BRCA2 mutation takes medication that lowers her ovarian cancer risk by 50 percent, her relative risk is then half of what it was compared to a woman with the mutation who doesn't take the medication.

MY STORY: I Assumed My Risk Was 100 Percent

Because I had atypical ductal hyperplasia (ADH), and my mother and both grandmothers had breast cancer, my breast surgeon said I had a very high risk of getting it too. I always thought I would somehow escape the breast cancer that ran in my family. Once I had ADH, I felt 100 percent certain

I would follow in my mother's and grandmothers' footsteps, so I had my
breasts removed. I found out later that I don't have a mutation. —KRIS

Knowing your lifetime risk for cancer has limited value when you're considering ways to manage your current risk. Addressing your risk over a specific timeframe is particularly important if you have a BRCA mutation, because you're more likely to be diagnosed with breast cancer before age 50. Understanding your incremental risk is also important when considering treatment options. A woman with sporadic breast cancer may choose breast-conserving surgery, knowing her risk for another tumor in ten years is just 10 percent. A woman with BRCA-related breast cancer might prefer mastectomy instead, because her risk of a second cancer over the same period is 30 percent.

EXPERT VIEW: Decade-by-Decade Risks

BY TIMOTHY R. REBBECK, PH.D.

The numbers in table 4 (see page 34) were derived from Johns Hopkins University researchers who combined nine studies that estimate cancer risks in BRCA mutation carriers. Combining studies to obtain composite risk estimates is a good way to provide more representative numbers when trying to understand risk variations across many small populations, as we see in BRCA carriers. Each study reported different risk results. These differences can be explained by how the studies were analyzed, which families and individuals were included, the total number of individuals who were included, and other factors. Table 4 supplies our best estimate of decade-by-decade and lifetime risk for BRCA1 and BRCA2 mutation carriers based on the aggregate of all nine studies. As we study more people with BRCA mutations, we gain a better idea of risk. It is important to remember that risk varies considerably between women: the estimates in table 4 represent an average risk across all populations. An individual's risk may be quite different from the average.

(continued)

Table 4. Average probability of developing breast or ovarian cancer

	Breast cancer risk with BRCA1 mutation (%)	Breast cancer risk with BRCA2 mutation (%)	Ovarian cancer risk with BRCA1 mutation (%)	Ovarian cancer risk with BRCA2 mutation (%)
By age 30	< 1	1	almost none	almost none
By age 40	2	10	4	2
By age 50	14	22	14	2
By age 60	32	36	28	10
By age 70	47	49	40	18
By age 80	57	49	40	18
Lifetime	64	56	55	31

Source: Chen S and Parmigiani G, "Meta-Analysis of BRCA1 and BRCA2 Penetrance," Journal of Clinical Oncology 25, no. 11 (2007): 1329–33.

THE FORCE (FACING OUR RISK OF CANCER EMPOWERED)
PERSPECTIVE: PUTTING MEDIA REPORTS INTO CONTEXT

Media stories about behaviors, foods, or other factors that raise or reduce cancer risk can be misleading if not put into proper context. Hearing that 1 in 10 women is obese by age 40 doesn't necessarily apply to you because your personal risk for obesity is different, depending on factors you can control: exercising regularly and eating balanced meals in proper proportions. Similarly, hearing that "exercise reduces breast cancer risk by 50 percent" doesn't necessarily mean your risk is half that of your couch-potato neighbor if you jog every day. The next time you hear one of these encouraging or scary reports, consider it with caution and talk to your doctor about how it may or may not affect you.

WHAT TO REMEMBER ABOUT RISK

- BRCA risk is a best guess based on current research.
- Risk is a moving target that changes throughout your lifetime.

- You can control certain risk factors; others you cannot.
- Your genes don't necessarily define your destiny. No matter what your risk, you can take steps to manage it.

LEARN MORE ABOUT RISK

The National Cancer Institute has an online Breast Cancer Risk Assessment Tool (www.cancer.gov/bcrisktool).

In the Family (inthefamily.kartemquin.com) is an award-winning documentary that follows previvor Joanna Rudnick and several families affected by hereditary breast and ovarian cancer.

Assess Your True Risk of Breast Cancer, by Patricia Kelley, Ph.D., is a comprehensive guide to cancer risk.

Reduce Your Cancer Risk: Twelve Steps to a Healthier Life, by Barbara Boughton and Mike Stefanek, Ph.D., explains risk-reducing strategies.

Chapter 4 Hereditary Cancer

What's Swimming in Your Gene Pool?

MUCH OF YOUR APPEARANCE results from traits you inherit from your parents. You can thank them for your cute dimples, stubby fingers, or widow's peak. These inherited characteristics are written into your DNA. You can pass them—and genetic mutations—on to your sons and daughters.

Mutations from Mom or Dad

All of us in the human race get half our genetic material from each parent. So it's equally possible to inherit a BRCA mutation from Mom or Dad. In fact, if we could identify every person with a BRCA mutation, we would find about half received their mutation from their father and half from their mother. If either of your parents has a BRCA mutation, you and each of your siblings have a 50 percent chance of inheriting it. Likewise, each of your children has the same 50 percent chance of inheriting your mutation and high cancer risk. Generally, children who don't inherit your mutation have average cancer risk.

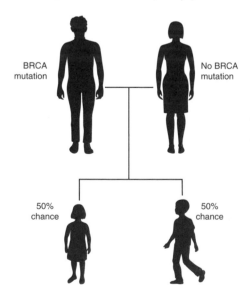

BRCA mutation

No BRCA mutation

50% chance

50% chance

Each child has a 50% chance of inheriting the mutation.

Probability of inheriting a mutation from one parent

Inheriting Multiple BRCA Mutations

While uncommon, it's possible to inherit mutations in both BRCA1 and BRCA2, especially if you're of Ashkenazi Jewish ethnicity. People with double mutations are believed to have risk for breast, ovarian, and fallopian cancer that is similar to individuals with BRCA1 mutations. Risk for melanoma, pancreatic cancer, prostate cancer, and male breast cancer is thought to be equivalent to someone with a BRCA2 mutation. If you have mutations in both BRCA genes, or you and your spouse each have a mutation, your risk of passing one or both mutations to your children is 75 percent. Embryos can grow with a double mutation in the BRCA2 gene, but they must have at least one working copy of BRCA1 to survive. Children who inherit a mutation in both copies of BRCA2—one mutation from each parent—develop Fanconi anemia (FA), a rare and serious childhood disorder characterized by bone marrow that doesn't produce enough blood cells. Several other genes are also linked with FA. Some children with this disorder have physical abnormalities such as altered skin pigment, deformed thumbs, a very small head size, or stunted growth. Other abnormalities in the heart, kidney, genitalia, or hearing may also develop. Blood abnormalities usually develop before age 12 and may include fatigue and paleness, bleeding or bruising, or susceptibility to infections from a low level of white blood cells.

Hidden Risk in the Family Tree

Sometimes it's difficult to determine whether a mutation runs in a family. Lifestyle choices, a small family size, having few female relatives, or having relatives who died early from other causes may obscure familial cancers. In some cases, family history may not be available. Many Ashkenazi Jewish families, for example, cannot trace their family history beyond the Holocaust. If you were adopted and don't know your family history, or your female relatives died before age 50 of unknown causes, a genetic counselor can help determine the likelihood that you inherited a mutation based on the information available.

Because either parent can pass a mutation to their children, ignoring Dad's side of the family can hide potential risk. Far fewer men than women with BRCA mutations develop cancer, potentially making indications of a mutation less obvious. Knowing the source of a mutation in your family can determine whether relatives on that side of the family may have the same mutation and associated high risk. A genetics expert can use your family history to try to determine whether a mutation came from your mother or father.

MY STORY: My Mutation Came from My Dad

Diagnosed with breast cancer, I thought I had no relevant family history. My father's first cousins had the disease; they were in their 60s and seemed like such distant relatives. I don't recall a single health form ever asking about my father's first cousin. After my diagnosis with breast cancer, I met with a genetic counselor who realized from my small family tree that my cancer likely came from my father's side. If he had more women on his side of the family, we may have seen more breast cancer. Sure enough, like my two cousins, I tested positive for a BRCA2 mutation.   —ELLYN

HBOC and Other Hereditary Cancer Syndromes

Hereditary cancer syndromes are caused by mutations that run in families and raise the risk of multiple cancers. BRCA mutations in a family cause hereditary breast and ovarian cancer (HBOC) syndrome, an inherited tendency for cancers of the breast, ovaries, fallopian tubes, pancreas, prostate, and skin. Several other cancer syndromes have been identified, each with a unique pattern of disease. Your family may have a hereditary cancer syndrome if multiple relatives have had certain types of cancers, including rare cancers; if the same cancer appears in more than one generation; or if cancers were diagnosed at a young age. One or two cases of the same types of cancer within a family—these days that includes many families—don't necessarily indicate a cancer

Table 5. Signs of HBOC within a family

Any blood relative with:	Ovarian or fallopian tube cancer at any age
	Breast cancer at age 50 or younger
	Breast cancer in both breasts at any age
	Both breast and ovarian cancer
	Male breast cancer
More than one relative on the same side of the family with:	Breast cancer
	Ovarian or fallopian tube cancer
	Prostate cancer
	Pancreatic cancer

syndrome. Any of the signs shown in table 5 may indicate that HBOC runs in the family.

Although HBOC is the most common cause of hereditary breast and ovarian cancer, inherited syndromes caused by mutations in other genes also increase the risk for these cancers.

Lynch Syndrome

Hereditary nonpolyposis colorectal cancer, also known as Lynch syndrome, increases risk for colon, uterine, and ovarian cancers. Women with Lynch syndrome have greater risk for ovarian cancer than other women, but less risk than someone who has a BRCA mutation. Caused by a mutation in one of several specific genes, Lynch syndrome is the most common hereditary cause of colon cancer, accounting for about 5 percent of all cases. If you have Lynch syndrome, you need regular screening at an early age—colonoscopy beginning between ages 20 and 25 is recommended—because you have a high risk for benign polyps that can develop into colon cancer if they're not removed during colonoscopy. Lynch syndrome may run in families in which a relative has been diagnosed with colorectal cancer more than once, when colorectal cancer or uterine cancer occurs in two successive generations in relatives age 50 or younger, or when three relatives have any of the cancers related to Lynch syndrome.

Cowden Syndrome

Cowden syndrome results from an inherited mutation in the PTEN tumor-suppressor gene. Even individuals who have no family history may develop the syndrome spontaneously. One in 200,000 people is estimated to have Cowden, with a risk of developing breast cancer as high as 50 percent.[1] Similar to individuals with BRCA mutations, diagnosis before age 50 may be more common. Only a small percentage of breast cancers are attributed to Cowden syndrome (it may be underdiagnosed). Having Cowden syndrome also ups the chance for other cancers, including thyroid (10 percent risk), endometrial (5 to 10 percent risk), and cancers of the kidney, colon, and skin (risk levels unknown). It's sometimes the underlying cause of otherwise unexplained cancers in families that test negative for a BRCA mutation.

Gene testing can identify this syndrome. It takes an experienced genetics expert to evaluate a family's unexplained cancers and determine if Cowden syndrome may be the culprit. Men and women with Cowden's have a higher-than-normal risk for both benign and cancerous growths including thyroid tumors; lesions of the skin, mouth, and lower digestive tract; and genital or uterine fibroids. Some studies have also linked PTEN mutations with melanoma and certain types of aggressive brain tumors. Other signs of this syndrome within a family are visible benign growths, such as lipomas (fatty lumps) or goiter (benign growth of the thyroid); polyps; hamartomas (benign masses); skin tags; fibrocystic breast changes; and intestinal polyps.

Li-Fraumeni Syndrome

Li-Fraumeni syndrome is caused by a rare inherited mutation in the P53 gene. This syndrome often causes childhood and adolescent cancers and carries a 50 to 80 percent risk of breast cancer between ages 15 and 44.[2] Individuals who have Li-Fraumeni often develop childhood cancers of the bone, soft tissue, adrenals, brain, stomach, and other organs.

Hereditary Diffuse Gastric Cancer Syndrome

Hereditary diffuse gastric cancer (HDGC) syndrome results from a mutation in the CDH1 gene. Little is known about HDGC. It can cause stomach cancers, often before age 40 (most gastric cancers in the general population are diagnosed after age 60). Women with an HDGC mutation have a 39 to 52 percent lifetime risk of developing lobular breast cancer.[3]

Peutz-Jeghers Syndrome

Peutz-Jeghers syndrome occurs from a mutation in the STK11 gene. Patients with this syndrome have elevated risk for breast and ovarian cancer, as well as cancer of the cervix, pancreas, and gastrointestinal tract. Children with Peutz-Jeghers often develop small dark freckles on the face, hands, feet, and anus that usually fade as they become teenagers. Thousands of polyps in the stomach and intestines are common in individuals with Peutz-Jeghers. It's a rare syndrome, and experts aren't sure how frequently it occurs.

Ataxia-Telangiectasia

Ataxia-telangiectasia (AT) is a rare disorder affecting only 1 in 100,000 births. It's believed to cause immune system cancers, including leukemia and lymphomas. Only individuals who inherit ATM gene mutations from both parents develop AT—but having a single mutation may predispose individuals to greater chance of developing breast cancer.

CDKN2A mutations

Mutations in the CDKN2A gene are also very rare. People who inherit this mutation have up to a 17 percent lifetime risk of pancreatic cancer and a 28 percent lifetime risk for melanoma.[4]

Plotting Your Genetic Pedigree

If your family has been affected by cancer, you've probably wondered about your own risk. A genetics expert can evaluate your family's pattern of disease to determine whether a mutation or hereditary cancer syndrome exists in your family, and whether you or a relative should consider genetic testing. First, you'll need to gather information to document your family's *pedigree*, or medical history. This document shows all your relatives, their relationship to you, and any diseases they've had. With this information, a genetic counselor can identify health patterns and determine your risk for inherited disease. Your pedigree can't predict your future health, but it can give you an insight your relatives never had: a peek into your future and the potential to change your fate by determining which diseases you're predisposed to develop.

Ideally, a genetics expert needs information from both sides of the family for three generations to determine whether a hereditary cancer pattern exists. So if possible, you'll need to collect information about your first-, second-, and third-degree biological relatives (see table 6).

Table 6. Gather information about three generations

First-degree relatives	Second-degree relatives	Third-degree relatives
siblings	half-siblings	cousins
children	uncles and aunts	great-grandparents
parents	grandparents	great-aunts and great-uncles
	grandchildren	
	nieces and nephews	

Generally, the closer the relationship between family members with cancer, the more significant the risk. Cancer in a first-degree relative more substantially affects your risk than cancer in a second-degree relative, which holds more significance than cancer in a third-degree relative. If possible, include information about all your blood relatives, including half-siblings (brothers or sisters with whom you share only one biological parent). Do not include step-relatives or in-laws: these are individuals who are a part of your family as a result of marriage; they don't share your bloodlines.

> **CLARIFYING YOUR CLAN**
>
> It can be confusing to label relatives, particularly in very large families with several cousins. Your first cousins are the children of your aunts and uncles (your parents' brothers and sisters). The children of your first cousins are your first cousins once removed. Your children and your cousins' children are second cousins to each other.

Discovering Your Medical Roots

The sooner you can collect your family history the better, because as each generation ages, the potential for information to become lost or forgotten increases. In some families, discussing cancer is taboo, particularly where breasts and ovaries are involved, and relatives may not want to divulge their medical histories. Emphasize how this information can help current and future family members manage their risk for disease. If individuals are uncomfortable talking about medical issues, ask if they're willing to provide written information. The more accurate the details, the more helpful the information will be. Family trees, bibles, and genealogy materials can be good data sources. If you were adopted, ask your adoptive parents. If possible, ask your birth parents about your medical history.

To build your pedigree, research and document as many of the following items as possible for each living and deceased relative:

- year of birth
- race and ethnicity
- any diagnosed cancer, whether or not it was the cause of death

- age at diagnosis
- age at death (If the exact age is unknown, estimate as accurately as possible. If your maternal aunt died between age 30 and 40, for example, but you don't know her exact age at the time, record "deceased in her 30s.")
- cause of death

MY STORY: Confronting a Legacy of Silence

My mother never discussed her breast cancer, her radical mastectomy, or her feelings. Only when I was 44 and facing my own breast cancer—thirty-three years later—did she share the details with me. As a child, I would sneak peeks at her satin prosthesis; it scared me to pieces. As a teenager, I wondered about my own risk, even then. I vowed to never keep my children in the dark about our family's cancer legacy. Now, it's my turn. I must find the right words to tell my children about others in our family who have developed cancers: my aunt, my cousin, my sister, and me. —LAUREN

EXPERT VIEW: Ignorance Is Not Bliss

BY MÓNICA ALVARADO, M.S., C.G.C.

Older relatives and those who were raised to believe that it is not acceptable to discuss cancer and other serious illnesses may be reluctant to share details about the family's cancer history. If you can help your relatives understand that sharing information about the family's pedigree is an important legacy, they may be more likely to cooperate. Here are some tips:

- If you can win the support of your family matriarchs and patriarchs, the most influential people in your family, other relatives will help you.
- Elderly relatives, your parents, and older siblings are more likely to know about your ancestors.
- Generally, women are much better than men at remembering health information. If you can identify key female relatives, ask them to help.

- Use other relatives as intermediaries if you are trying to get information from someone you do not know well.
- If you have amateur genealogists in your family, they may have already collected the family history.
- Take advantage of family events such as weddings, reunions, and funerals to contact relatives.
- Use additional resources like family diaries, newspaper clippings, public records, public libraries and archives, books, and pamphlets for additional suggestions.
- Be sensitive to the fact that adoption, divorce, drug abuse, suicide, and other topics may be difficult to discuss. Acknowledge the fact, but try to explain why it's important to have the most accurate history available.

If you can, be sure to distinctly note the type of cancer someone had. If Aunt Sarah says her mother had brain cancer, try to determine whether it was truly brain cancer or breast cancer that metastasized to the brain, if that information is available. Identifying gynecologic cancers can also be confusing. Was your grandmother's abdominal condition really ovarian cancer? If possible, find out whether someone's "female" disease was cancer of the ovaries, uterus, cervix, or other reproductive organ.

You can gather all your information before creating your pedigree or create it as you discover information. The U.S. Department of Health and Human Services (https://familyhistory.hhs.gov) provides easy online tools for both methods. "My Family Health Portrait" produces a chart of your family medical history based on your input. Just hop online and follow the prompts. If someone in your family has already created a pedigree, most or all of the work will be done for you. Just make sure it's up to date and reflects all the specific information you need. If it doesn't, make it as comprehensive as you can. Take very good care of your pedigree. Keep a copy in a safety deposit box, and if the document is stored on your computer, be sure to make a backup copy. Update it whenever a birth, death, or diagnosis occurs in the family.

Sample family pedigree

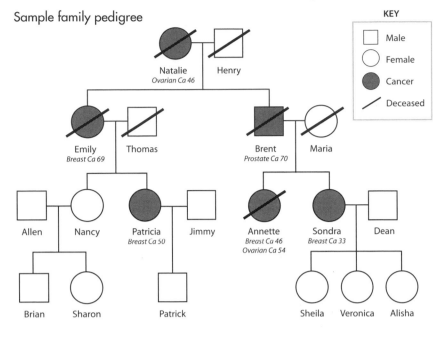

KEY

- ☐ Male
- ◯ Female
- ⬤ Cancer
- ╱ Deceased

WHAT TO REMEMBER ABOUT HEREDITARY CANCER RISK

- BRCA mutations can be inherited from your mother or father.
- On average, half of one's children will inherit a parent's BRCA mutation.
- Hereditary cancer syndromes raise the risk for multiple cancers.
- An accurate family pedigree is necessary to identify patterns of inherited disease.

LEARN MORE ABOUT HEREDITARY CANCER

Facing Our Risk of Cancer Empowered (www.facingourrisk.org) provides information, networking, and support for individuals at high risk for hereditary breast and ovarian cancer.

PART TWO ASSESSING YOUR RISK

Chapter 5   Genetic Counseling

AS GENETIC SCIENCE brings us closer to personalized medicine, the need for specialized health care is increasing. One such specialty is genetic counseling, the process of evaluating an individual's personal and family medical history to assess cancer risk and customize a plan for risk management or treatment. This well-established field is evolving as new genetic discoveries are made.

The Value of Counseling

If you suspect that cancer runs in your family, have signs of a hereditary cancer syndrome, or think you should be tested for a BRCA mutation, you'll benefit from talking with a genetic counselor, who will provide the following services:

- Identify patterns of inherited cancer that run in your family.
- Determine which family members, if any, should consider genetic testing, and in what order.
- Discuss the benefits and limitations of genetic testing for you and your family to help you decide if testing is right for you.
- Decide which genetic test is most appropriate.
- Interpret test results and explain what they mean for you and your family.
- Estimate your cancer risk, whether or not you have a BRCA mutation.
- Discuss how to manage and reduce your cancer risk.
- Explain how a mutation affects your risk of another cancer or your treatment options (if you've been diagnosed with cancer).

Dealing with cancer in the family is difficult. Learning it's heredi-tary can be even more upsetting. A genetic counselor is trained and experienced in disease-related genetics and psychosocial counseling. She can translate what may seem to be incomprehensible concepts into clear terms and meaningful estimates of your risk, and help you and your family cope with the information. Genetic counselors don't try to persuade you to be tested or tell you what to do; they provide invaluable input to help you make informed decisions and reduce the likelihood that you or your relatives will hear, "You have cancer."

The National Comprehensive Cancer Network (NCCN)—a consor-tium of the nation's leading cancer experts who dictate standard-of-care guidelines in oncology—and most other medical organizations recom-mend genetic counseling before genetic testing. It's a critical first step, even if you decide not to be tested. If you are tested, it may determine whether your insurance will cover the cost.

MY STORY: Don't Try This—Genetic Testing without Counseling

I received my genetic test results without the benefit of a genetic counselor because I didn't know there was such a thing! A nurse took my family his-tory, read the options on the brochure, and told me I would probably test positive. No one ever asked me why I wanted to be tested or what I would do with the results. Without any preparation, I was informed that I was positive. I met with a group of doctors, who told me I needed to have bilat-eral mastectomies right away. No one wanted to answer questions about my risk, my options, or what this test result meant for my family. It is cruel to receive results in this way, then be sent on your way and wished good luck. I never felt so alone in my life.   —ALICE

What to Expect from the Process

The NCCN recommends guidelines for referring individuals for BRCA testing. The criteria are not always straightforward, however, and no risk-assessment model by itself can replace an evaluation by a genetics expert. After an in-depth discussion of your medical history and pedigree, your counselor will use computerized programs, national guidelines, and her expertise to determine whether you or other relatives would likely benefit from genetic testing.

- If the cancer in a family suggests a sporadic pattern with no evidence of inherited disease, genetic testing is not recommended.
- If your pedigree shows evidence of an inherited syndrome or pattern of cancer for which a genetic test is available, testing is recommended.

If you decide to be tested, your counselor will explain the process and arrange for a blood or mouth rinse sample to be sent to the testing laboratory. After your test, she'll provide a copy of your results and explain how they affect your risk of breast, ovarian, or other cancers. She'll also discuss your risk management options. If you're interested, she can inform you of screening, prevention, or treatment research studies for which you may be eligible. If you've already been tested for a mutation without the benefit of prior counseling, a genetics expert can provide this same level of post-testing information and support. Based on your family pedigree, she'll identify other family members who might also benefit from genetic counseling and testing and provide contact

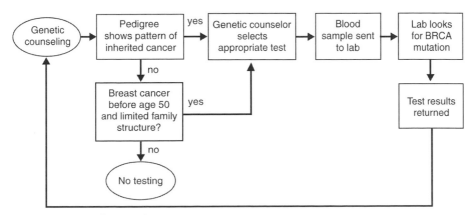

Genetic counseling and testing process

information for an expert in their area. If your test was negative, your counselor may recommend other genetic tests to help further define the cause of the cancer in your family.

Genetic counseling centers that provide in-person services may require separate visits for counseling, testing, and receiving results. For individuals who decide to pursue testing, most centers now draw a blood sample during the first counseling session, thereby saving the patient another visit, and then provide test results either over the phone or during another appointment. Some genetic counselors require a separate visit for the blood sample, so it's a good idea to ask about a center's process when you make your appointment.

Why You Need an Expert to Unravel Your Genetic History

When a stubborn rash refuses to go away, you see a dermatologist. When cancer is diagnosed, you consult with an oncologist. Likewise, when you want to know if your family has a hereditary pattern of disease or learn about your risk for cancer, you need a genetics professional. Your primary physician, gynecologist, or other clinician may be skilled and compassionate professionals, but if they don't have current and advanced genetics training and expertise— some nurses and other healthcare providers do—and the time to provide a detailed consultation, they're not the best source to determine whether you should be tested, to interpret your results, or to assess your overall risk.

At best, risk assessment is a delicate and ambiguous process with hereditary red flags that aren't always obvious, and it

RISK ASSESSMENT FOR ASIAN WOMEN

The most commonly used BRCA risk-assessment models accurately identify most women who might benefit from genetic testing, but in the past, they underestimated Asian women's chance of carrying a BRCA mutation. If you're Asian and have cancer in your family, speak with a genetic counselor to see if BRCA testing is beneficial.

Source: Kurian AW, et al., "Performance of BRCA1/2 Mutation Prediction Models in Asian Americans," *Journal of Clinical Oncology* 26, no. 29 (2008): 4752–58.

takes particular skill and training to figure them all out. Take another look at the bulleted items at the beginning of this chapter that list the range of services genetic counselors provide. Most doctors aren't trained to do all this. Skilled interpreters of risk, counselors are genetic gurus who represent the human side of science and can help you navigate the entire counseling-testing process. They know how stressful test results can be, and they're sensitive to your concerns and fears. By answering and probably anticipating your questions, a genetic counselor will put your test results into proper perspective and present medical options so that you can make informed decisions about your health care, reduce your risk (whether you test positive for a mutation or not), and move on with your life.

One final word about genetic counselors: stay in touch. As genetic research progresses, we're learning more about BRCA mutations and other causes of hereditary cancer, so it's a good idea to revisit your status each year—or when any new case of cancer is diagnosed in the family—with your genetic counselor. When new mutations are discovered, she'll continue to be an invaluable resource.

EXPERT VIEW: Experience Counts

BY JANA PRUSKI-CLARK, M.P.H., M.S., C.G.C.

Until people go through the process of genetic counseling with a trained genetics professional, they may consider genetic testing to be a clear-cut blood test that will tell them if they have "the breast cancer gene" or not. But genetic testing is more than just a blood test. It offers many benefits, providing information about your medical options for cancer screening, risk reduction, and treatment. It also has limitations, including those related to cost, insurance coverage, privacy, and interpretation of results, especially when results are uncertain or uninformative. Both positive and negative results can have psychological impact; despite all of our medical advances, it's never easy to hear that you're at increased risk for cancer.

As genetic counselors, we know that testing involves individuals yet affects entire families: Who else should be tested? Do relatives want to know your

(continued)

results? What, how, and when do you tell your kids? Genetic counselors are trained to help you answer these questions as they support you and your family throughout the entire process. And although we may not have walked in your shoes, we've walked alongside others with cancer in the family, and we can share that knowledge with you.

MY STORY: My Age Was a Red Flag

I was shocked to be diagnosed at age 33 because I was the first in my family with breast cancer. The only other cancer I knew of was my dad's mother, who died young of "kidney cancer" decades earlier. Eight months after completing treatment, I read an article about the family link between breast and ovarian cancer. It stated that BRCA mutations were more common in younger women with breast cancer and in people of Ashkenazi Jewish descent. That was me. I realized my grandmother's kidney cancer may have been advanced ovarian cancer. Genetic counseling and testing confirmed I had a BRCA2 mutation. I wish my doctors had referred me to a genetics expert when I was diagnosed; had I known of my BRCA status then, I would have made different surgical choices. —SUE

Deciding Who Should Test First

Anyone with a family history of breast or ovarian cancer can benefit from genetic counseling; only some will benefit from genetic testing, because most people who are tested have negative results. Even though you may be anxious to find out if you have a BRCA mutation, particularly if a close relative has been diagnosed with breast or ovarian cancer, it may make more sense (and prove more valuable to you and your family) to first test a relative. Genetic testing is most reliable when it begins with a family member who has been diagnosed with cancer and has the highest likelihood of testing positive. Your pedigree will help a genetic counselor determine who this should be. Then, if that family member tests positive, others can be tested for the same mutation. If you've never had cancer, but your maternal aunt had ovarian cancer or young-onset breast cancer, testing her first is more informative. If she tests positive for a BRCA abnormality, your mother could be tested for the same mutation. If she also has the mutation, you and your siblings can be tested. If your mother's test shows no known mutation, there's no point in testing you or your siblings for your aunt's mutation (your mother can't give you a mutation she doesn't have). You might want to be tested if your mother is no longer living, because there's no way to know if she had the mutation.

If more than one relative has had cancer, it's best to first test whoever was diagnosed with breast cancer at the earliest age or with a less common cancer (ovarian, fallopian tube, or pancreatic cancer). If your sister Beth had breast cancer at age 50, and your sister Jane had ovarian cancer at age 48, it may be best to first test Jane, in case Beth's breast cancer was sporadic. If Jane tests positive, other relatives who haven't had cancer can then be tested for her mutation.

When it's not possible to begin testing with a cancer survivor in the family, testing a relative who hasn't had cancer is more likely to produce an inconclusive result that can create a false sense of security. She may have a known mutation in a different gene or in a gene we don't know about today and therefore don't know how to find. In this case, a genetic counselor can identify the best candidate to begin the testing process and determine whether others in the family should be tested. This doesn't mean you shouldn't have genetic testing. It can, however, make interpretation of a negative test result more confusing. If both sides of the family show a history of cancer, individuals on both sides

SEVEN QUESTIONS FOR YOUR
GENETIC COUNSELOR

1. Does my family history show a pattern of inherited disease?
2. Should I be tested to see if I've inherited a predisposition to disease?
3. For which mutations will I be tested?
4. How reliable are the test results?
5. What does the test mean for me and my family members?
6. What are my options if I test positive?
7. Will my test results change my treatment? (If you're currently being treated for cancer.)

should see a genetic counselor. If your mother tests negative and your father's pedigree shows a history of cancer, his family may also benefit from genetic counseling. These are complex issues, which is why expert involvement is so valuable.

INSURANCE AND PAYMENT ISSUES

Genetic counseling is considered a preventive service that is covered by most types of health insurance with no out-of-pocket costs. Even when your insurance would otherwise cover the cost of counseling, circumstances may compel you to pay for these services yourself. If your in-network genetic counselor can't see you as soon as you'd like, for example, you may decide to pay out-of-pocket to see a counselor outside your plan sooner. Genetic counselors are familiar with state and federal laws regarding information and discrimination, so they can address your concerns about the privacy and confidentiality of your genetic information.

THE FORCE PERSPECTIVE: WHEN COUNSELING DOESN'T HAPPEN

We see many instances where lack of genetic counseling leads to harm. One FORCE member and two of her siblings who received genetic testing through a healthcare provider weren't offered and didn't receive prior genetic counseling. All three were told their BRCA test was positive. Considering herself at high risk for breast and ovarian cancer, the woman had her healthy ovaries removed. When a relative was later tested for the same mutation, her genetic counselor determined the FORCE member's test result was, in fact, not positive—the misinformation resulted in her unnecessary, irreversible surgery and testing (and related anxiety and cost) her siblings didn't need.

Another FORCE member was advised by her physician to be tested after a breast cancer diagnosis. She decided to have bilateral mastectomies if the test showed she carried a BRCA mutation. When her test came back negative, she chose lumpectomy and radiation to treat her cancer, thinking she had average risk for a subsequent cancer. After her surgery, an oncologist discovered that the woman had been told to complete her own paperwork for the BRCA test—something usually done by a genetic counselor; in the process, she unknowingly ordered the wrong test and acted on the wrong result.

WHAT TO REMEMBER ABOUT GENETIC COUNSELING

A genetics expert is the best resource to:
- determine whether cancer runs in your family.
- advise if you or someone else in the family can benefit from genetic testing.
- decide which test is most appropriate and explain your test results.
- provide updated information about mutations and risk.

LEARN MORE ABOUT GENETIC COUNSELING

The National Society of Genetic Counselors (www.nsgc.org) maintains a searchable directory of counselors by state and area of expertise.

The National Cancer Institute (www.cancer.gov/cancertopics/genetics /directory) provides an online list of healthcare providers who offer genetic counseling as well as their certification credentials.

Informed Medical Decisions (www.informedmedicaldecisions.com or 800-975-4819) provides genetic counseling by telephone with board-certified counselors. (One of this book's authors, Dr. Rebecca Sutphen, is chief medical officer of this company.)

Chapter 6 Genetic Testing

Facing Your Hereditary Horoscope

IT'S AN AGE-OLD QUESTION: If you could see into your future, would you want to? A better question might be: If you could change your potentially high-risk destiny, would you?

Hundreds of predictive blood and tissue tests can reveal whether you're an above-average candidate for disease, and more are quickly becoming available. Still, genetic testing for cancer risk isn't a true crystal ball. The glimpse it gives isn't a guarantee that you'll get cancer, but it can tell you if your risk is steep. So why explore your cancer risk when there are no guarantees? Because testing gives you and your family the chance to reshape your future, particularly if you have a risk-raising mutation, by clarifying your choices: wait and see what happens, screen to detect cancer early, or pre-emptively act to reduce your odds of developing breast or ovarian cancer.

If you decide to pursue BRCA testing after counseling, a small needle prick or a mouth rinse begins the testing process. Your sample will be sent to Myriad Genetics, a commercial laboratory, where a technician will separate your BRCA genes from the rest of your DNA and scan them for abnormalities. Results are forwarded to the healthcare professional who ordered the test, usually in two to three weeks or longer if you live outside the country.

Which Test Is Right for You?

Myriad's BRACAnalysis test explores segments of the BRCA genes where we expect to find a mutation. Current tests locate most (not all) cancer-causing mutations in the BRCA genes. Scientists know that others exist, but we can test only for those we know about. It's like space exploration: we know how to navigate to Mars, yet we haven't a clue about traveling to other solar systems—even though we know they're out there somewhere.

Hereditary syndromes caused by less common mutations in other genes require different testing procedures from different labs. Your genetic counselor can explain whether it makes sense for you to pursue these. Most BRCA tests involve one of three types:

1. Full-sequencing tests look for abnormalities in BRCA1 and BRCA2. This is a first step when no one else in the family has been tested, or if those already tested had negative results and a mutation is still suspected.
2. Single-site tests search for a specific mutation already identified in the family.
3. Multisite tests search for the three most common BRCA founder mutations in people of Ashkenazi Jewish descent. These mutations have been passed from generation to generation over hundreds of years. Among Ashkenazi, 90 percent of all BRCA abnormalities are one of three founder mutations: 185delAG mutation in BRCA1, 5382insC mutation in BRCA1, or 6174delT mutation in BRCA2.

BRCA testing comes with a high price tag, from about $400 to $4,000, depending on the test. Full sequencing is more expensive than other tests because it examines hundreds of areas on BRCA1 and BRCA2. Single-site and multisite tests evaluate only a few areas of the BRCA genes and are less expensive. Myriad also offers the BRACAnalysis Rearrangement Test (BART), an additional diagnostic that looks for less common BRCA mutations known as *large rearrangements*. BART is run at no charge on all samples for breast and ovarian cancer survivors who meet

ARE YOU ASHKENAZI?

Eighty percent of the world's Jewish population has roots in medieval Germany (Ashkenaz is the Hebrew word for Germany) and later dispersed throughout Hungary, Poland, Russia, and Eastern Europe. The remaining 20 percent are Sephardic groups, with ancestors from Spain, Portugal, North Africa, and the Middle East, who don't usually carry Ashkenazi founder mutations. Most of America's 6 million Jewish individuals are Ashkenazi.

Myriad's family history criteria. The test, which may not be covered by insurance, can be ordered separately if you don't meet the criteria or if you had a standard BRACAnalysis test prior to August 2006. Results are provided in about two weeks. A genetic counselor can help you decide if BART is appropriate for you or someone in your family.

MY STORY: What's the Point in Knowing?

I remember talking with my father about genetic testing, and he asked, "What is the point in knowing?" I think he believed the knowledge would just cause me suffering; better to wait for your fate and be surprised by it than suffer with the knowledge that it was coming. Perhaps this was part of his pragmatism or part of his growing up in the Philippines, where resources were limited—you just played the cards you were dealt. At that time, my father didn't know there was something you could do if you had positive test results. Once he knew I could take actions like surgeries to reduce my risk, and that what I got in return was the opportunity to avoid cancer, he and my mother told me that testing was the bravest thing I'd ever done for myself and for those who love me. —GRACE

Powerful, Yet Imperfect

BRCA testing isn't perfect, and like most things in life, it has advantages and disadvantages. On the beneficial side, testing clarifies cancer risk and empowers you to make decisions about current and future medical options. Your testing may help to inform others in your family about their hereditary cancer risk as well. On the other hand, testing can be complicated. It doesn't always provide a simple "yes" or "no" about hereditary cancer risk. Learning you have a BRCA mutation can quickly turn your otherwise rosy world topsy-turvy. You may feel helpless, uncertain about your future, overwhelmed, and even guilty about the chance of passing your mutation to your children.

EXPERT VIEW: Should Your Children Be Tested?

BY KENNETH P. TERCYAK, PH.D.

This is a common question for women and men who test positive for an alteration in BRCA1 or BRCA2, and sometimes children ask whether they can be tested. Medical organizations don't endorse BRCA testing for children under age 18, for several reasons. Children that young don't have the capacity to make an informed choice about testing and may not appreciate the long-lasting reach of the information, and they may suffer harm (psychological or otherwise) or regret their decision later on. If testing showed they had a mutation, no known action taken before age 18 would improve their risk for cancer.

You may, however, talk openly with your children about your own testing experiences—why you made a particular choice, what it means for you, and when testing might be age appropriate for them. Be open and honest about what you know and how you feel. This can be an opportunity to teach your children about healthy lifestyles, ways to prevent cancer, and available resources such as FORCE. It may also be comforting for children to know that researchers are working hard to find ways to prevent cancer, and new breakthroughs can and do happen.

Issues for Survivors and Women in Treatment

If you have breast cancer and your family history makes you a candidate for genetic testing, your test results may influence your decisions about treatment and future screening. For an additional cost, BRCA tests can be expedited for newly diagnosed individuals for whom test results may affect treatment choices.

If you have unilateral breast cancer and were planning to have breast-conserving lumpectomy with radiation, knowing you have a BRCA mutation might change your mind. For many women with sporadic cancer, breast-conserving lumpectomy followed by radiation may be as effective as mastectomy for treating breast cancer. High-risk women often choose *bilateral mastectomy* (removal of both breasts) instead to avoid radiation or to address their greater chance (compared to women with sporadic cancer) of developing a new cancer in the same or opposite breast. If you prefer breast conservation, intensive screening (discussed in chapter 8) may catch a future breast cancer at an early stage, and chemoprevention medications can reduce your risk (chapter 9). You would also want to address your higher chance for ovarian cancer with chemoprevention, surveillance, or surgery (chapter 12).

Testing for Young Survivors with Little or No Family History

Most risk-assessment models look for multiple cases of cancer in a family to help experts determine whether individuals should be tested for a mutation. But some women have few female relatives. Researchers define a *limited family structure* as having only one or no close female relatives older than 45. An enlightening study at City of Hope found that women in this category who had no family history and were diagnosed with breast cancer before age 50 were more likely to have a mutation than women with larger families and no family history of cancer.[1] Based on this study, experts recommend genetic counseling for any woman who develops breast cancer before age 50, whether or not she has a family history of the disease.

DNA BANKING

Banking DNA allows people to preserve their genes for future testing. An individual's DNA can be extracted from a sample of blood, cheek swab, or tissue (for example, leftover tumor tissue from surgery) for a modest price and can be easily stored. That individual then controls when and how the sample is used. DNA banking is an option for people who decide they don't want genetic testing now but would like to make their DNA available if relatives want that information in the future. Sometimes elderly or terminally ill people bank their DNA for later testing if relatives want to find out whether there is a mutation in the family. Members of families that have many cancers but no identified BRCA or other mutation might bank their DNA for testing when researchers discover new genes and mutations that cause cancer. Your genetic counselor can provide more information and help you find appropriate and confidential banking resources.

INSURANCE, PAYMENT, AND PRIVACY ISSUES

Most insurance plans, including Medicare, cover the cost of genetic testing as medically necessary if you meet certain criteria, and you make any required co-payment or deductible. Medicare covers the cost of testing only for people who have already been diagnosed with cancer. Your insurance company may require a letter from your genetic counselor or referring physician stating the medical necessity of the test. Payment may be denied for testing relatives who don't have cancer or who aren't considered to be at high risk. Insurance companies may deny claims for incorrect or inappropriate tests—another good reason to see a genetic counselor before you're tested. If your healthcare professional orders a test without first getting insurance company approval, you could get stuck with the bill. A genetics expert can determine whether your health plan covers testing and help you obtain preauthorization.

If you don't have insurance or you're denied coverage and can't afford testing, limited financial assistance is available. Myriad's Reimbursement Assistance Program offers testing at no charge if you meet certain medical and financial criteria and have no health insurance. Some state Medicaid programs currently cover BRACAnalysis if you meet eligibility criteria. A genetics expert can help determine if you do. The National Gene Test Fund (www.ngtf.org) underwrites the cost for eligible individuals, and FORCE maintains a national database of facilities that offer free testing and related services. Some research studies offer opportunities for genetic testing to people who meet certain criteria; test results may take five or six months.

People often fear genetic discrimination based on their test results, yet few documented cases of such an occurrence exist. If you haven't been diagnosed with a disease for which you are genetically predisposed, the Genetic Information Nondiscrimination Act (GINA) prohibits health insurers and employers from discriminating against you based on your test results or simply because you have a BRCA mutation. Health insurers cannot deny coverage, define terms of coverage, or set your premiums

(continued)

based on your genetic information. Employers cannot use your genetic information for hiring, firing, promotions, or any other decisions regarding your terms of employment. If you've already had cancer and you test positive for a BRCA mutation, GINA doesn't prevent insurance companies from viewing your diagnosis as pre-existing, but they can't use the test and your high risk for a new cancer as a basis for discrimination. Several states also have laws that protect against genetic discrimination; some offer more protection than GINA. The law doesn't apply to members of the military. No similar federal laws prevent discrimination for life, disability, or long-term care insurance. Some people apply for these plans before they have genetic testing.

If you've already been diagnosed, the Health Insurance Portability and Accountability Act (HIPAA) requires healthcare professionals to notify you about your privacy rights, and in most instances, requires your permission before your health information may be shared. Your genetic test results are kept in confidence as part of your medical record. If you're nervous about privacy, some healthcare providers allow you to submit your sample under an anonymous name; in this case, you'll have to pay for the test yourself. You may need to disclose your test results anyway if you want your insurance company to pay for MRIs, preventive surgery, or other procedures resulting from a positive test.

While health insurers may deny coverage or increase premiums for an entire insured group, HIPAA prohibits insurers from denying or canceling coverage, or raising rates for an individual within the group because of a pre-existing condition. (It doesn't apply to individual health policies or coverage for life or disability insurance.) When applying for a new healthcare policy, insurers may exclude coverage for a pre-existing condition for which you've seen a physician in the past six months. They may also delay coverage of your existing condition (while providing coverage for other health issues), depending on the length of your previous healthcare policy.

Pre-existing conditions won't be an issue for much longer. As part of sweeping healthcare reform passed in 2010, the Patient Protection and Affordable Care Act prohibits group plans from denying coverage or excluding benefits due to a pre-existing condition. The law already applies to children under age 19; it becomes effective for adults in 2014. At that time, insurance plans will no longer be allowed to charge higher premiums for individuals with pre-existing conditions. Until then, the federally mandated Pre-Existing Condition Insurance Plan program provides health coverage to people who haven't had health insurance for at least the last six months and who have been unable to obtain insurance from private insurance companies because of a pre-existing condition.

THE FORCE PERSPECTIVE: PUBLIC PERCEPTION OF GENETIC DISCRIMINATION

Before GINA, some people refused testing for fear of genetic discrimination. When we surveyed 805 people about genetic discrimination and GINA, we found that:

- many people are unaware of federal laws that protect against genetic discrimination in health insurance and employment.
- even among people who are aware of the laws, some still express worry about discrimination by insurance companies and employers.
- healthcare providers often don't discuss discrimination or legal protections with patients who have genetic testing.

WHAT TO REMEMBER ABOUT GENETIC TESTING

- Genetic testing indicates whether you've inherited a mutation and have greater risk for cancer. It doesn't determine whether you have cancer now or predict if you'll definitely develop it later.
- BRCA mutations have been found in people of every ethnicity, but they occur more frequently in people of Ashkenazi Jewish heritage.
- If you tested negative for a mutation prior to August 1, 2006, you may benefit from BART if you have a strong family history.
- Knowing your BRCA status may change your decisions about breast cancer treatment and future screening or prevention.

LEARN MORE ABOUT GENETIC TESTING

A genetic counselor is your best resource about testing. Find a counselor online (www.nsgc.org or www.informedmedicaldecisions.com. One of this book's authors, Dr. Rebecca Sutphen, is chief medical officer of Informed Medical Decisions).

FORCE (www.facingourrisk.org) provides information about financial assistance for genetic testing. (From the "Information and Research" menu, click on "Finding Health Care," then "Financial Help.")

The Genetic Information Nondiscrimination Act website (www .ginahelp.org) is a comprehensive resource about the law and how it protects you.

Chapter 7 Decoding Your Test Results

THE WAIT IS OVER. You've wondered, worried, and anxiously anticipated your test results. Now you're about to find out whether you're indeed at high risk or if you can perhaps breathe a sigh of relief. But that piece of paper in your hand may not completely clarify your cancer risk. It's important to speak with a genetics expert about your results, no matter what they are, so that you understand the implications for you and other family members. BRCA testing produces three categories of results: "positive for a deleterious mutation," "no mutation detected," or a "variant of uncertain significance." Here's a review of all three.

Life, Interrupted: It's Positive

It's probably the last thing you want to hear: *positive for a deleterious mutation* means you have a known mutation in BRCA1 or BRCA2. This result also means:

- You inherited a genetic mutation from one of your parents.
- You have increased risk for breast, ovarian, and other cancers.
- Your biological siblings have a 50 percent chance of having the same mutation.
- Your cousins, aunts, uncles, and other blood relatives (on the side of the family from which you inherited the mutation) may have the same mutation.
- Your biological children have a 50 percent chance of inheriting your mutation.

Testing positive for a BRCA mutation means you have tough decisions ahead: what should you do with the knowledge that your lifetime risk of developing breast and ovarian cancer is very high? Subsequent chapters describe your options: increased surveillance, medication to lower your risk, or prophylactic surgery. If you're the first in your family to test positive, your relatives can be tested for the same mutation at a lower cost.

Good News! You're a True Negative

A negative result means your test didn't find the specific BRCA mutations it was looking for. If you haven't had cancer, a family member already tested positive for a mutation, and your single-site test shows *no mutation detected*, you're considered a true negative. You didn't inherit the family mutation, and you therefore can't pass it on to your children. Your cancer risk is likely the same as anyone in the general population, with a remote possibility that you could have a different mutation. Other strong genetic or environmental factors may be affecting the cancer risk in your family. You should begin or continue routine screening as recommended by your doctor and genetic counselor.

When No Might Mean Maybe

If your result shows *no mutation detected*, it means your test showed no evidence of known BRCA mutations. In one way, that's wonderful news. However, you might have a different mutation that requires a separate test, is in a different gene, or is one that scientists don't know about yet. Having a negative test result doesn't always mean you have average risk. It might imply something else, depending on your family history and the type of test you had:

- If several people in your family have cancer but test negative, something other than a BRCA mutation may be the cause. The cancer could be caused by a different hereditary syndrome or an unknown mutation. It might be a combination of gene changes or a common behavior or environmental exposure.

- If you're the first in your family to have genetic testing, and you were tested for one of the three Ashkenazi founder mutations, *no mutation detected* means you have none of them. However, you might have a high risk for breast and ovarian cancer because of a different mutation, especially if both sides of your family have a history of either disease. If you're of Ashkenazi descent, you may have a less common mutation in BRCA1 or BRCA2 that isn't included in the founder test. A genetic counselor can explain if you or a family member might benefit from a more comprehensive, full-sequence gene test that would broadly search for other BRCA mutations.

- If your family has no known mutation and you haven't had cancer, the next step may be testing a relative who has been diagnosed with breast or ovarian cancer. You may still be at high risk due to an unknown mutation or a mutation that wasn't included in your test, especially if your family has a strong history of breast or ovarian cancer.

If any of these describe your situation, you should be screened closely and stay in touch with your genetics expert for new information and additional tests.

MY STORY: Acting on My Test Results

Eight of ten women in the three generations before me had breast cancer, so I was pretty sure if I had a BRCA mutation, my odds of developing breast cancer were close to 100 percent. My father's family has a strong history of breast cancer that includes four of his six sisters (three diagnosed before menopause), two aunts (one before menopause), and both great-aunts, who were likely premenopausal when diagnosed. After I found out about my BRCA2 mutation on my 35th birthday, I was on the operating table just six months later having bilateral mastectomies. —BETHANY

Genetic Variants

Small genetic changes aren't always significant—a slight variation may be the difference between brown and green eyes but doesn't affect eye function. The same is true with BRCA mutations. Some gene changes cause increased risk, while others don't. About 1 percent of the general population has genetic changes that don't significantly raise their risk for disease. A test result of *genetic variant, favor polymorphism* means you have one of these changes in BRCA1 or BRCA2 that is assumed not to raise cancer risk. A test result of *genetic variant, favor deleterious* means you have a gene change that is strongly suspected although not proved to be associated with hereditary cancer. When a test identifies a gene change but can't determine whether it raises cancer risk, the result is known as a *variant of uncertain significance* (VUS).

When a test result shows a VUS, it means a change was recognized in a BRCA gene, but whether it increases cancer risk is unknown. Over time, as more people are tested and more is known about individual variants, a VUS may be reclassified as harmful (BRCA positive) or harmless (BRCA negative). If your test shows you have a VUS, recommended cancer screenings and risk management will be based on your personal and family medical history. These recommendations may be different from those advised for people with different test results or those in the general population. Stay in contact with your genetics specialist, so you'll know if researchers discover new information that reclassifies your variant.

Variants of uncertain significance are considered to be *uninformative tests* because they don't provide a clear answer about a person's cancer risk. Compared to Caucasians, African Americans more often have uninformative genetic test results, especially a VUS.

When a family has a strong history of cancer and a family member's test shows a VUS, there may be several possible explanations:

- The VUS is really a harmful mutation, but not enough research exists to conclude that it's deleterious.
- The VUS is not harmful, and cancers that run in the family are caused

by a mutation in a different gene or in an unknown gene for which there is no available test.

- The VUS is not harmful, and cancers that run in the family are due to environmental factors or a combination of genetic and environmental factors.

EXPERT VIEW: Functional Analysis of Unclassified Variants

BY SUSAN M. DOMCHEK, M.D.

Classifying variants of unknown significance as benign (harmless) or deleterious (harmful) is a constantly evolving process. It includes careful examination of a patient's personal and family history, tracking the VUS in affected family members, and determining whether it has also been seen with a known deleterious mutation. This can be time consuming, taking years to reclassify variants.

New techniques are being developed to classify a variant as harmless or harmful depending on whether it affects the function of the gene. One such technique involves observing whether a copy of a gene with the VUS restores function when it's placed into laboratory mice who don't have a normal working BRCA gene. It's an expensive process but one that may provide a quicker method of determining if a VUS is deleterious or harmless.

Now What? Implications for You and Your Family

We all react differently, yet very often, a positive result may cause strong emotions: sadness, fear, worry, guilt, and even relief about finally knowing why cancer runs in the family. Sometimes an expected positive test result creates unanticipated reactions. You now have some difficult decisions to make about managing your risk. You'll also need to consider what to tell other family members who'll want to determine their own risk.

HOW ACCURATE IS YOUR TEST?

BRCA testing technology is highly accurate for known mutations. Testing is performed according to federal quality standards to ensure the accuracy, reliability, and timeliness of patient test results and is subject to routine regulatory inspections at the state and national levels.

If you have a negative test result, you may be elated. Perhaps you feel a sense of renewed commitment to lower your risk even further. Some women react differently. Escaping a BRCA mutation may create feelings of guilt if a sister, parent, or other close relative tests positive. Others may have a false sense of security, feeling that their negative test exempts them from regular mammograms and breast exams, which of course it doesn't. No matter what your test turned up, your genetic counselor can help demystify test terminology, put your risk into perspective, and help you sort out your feelings and consider your next step.

MY STORY: Why My Sister and Not Me?

When my sister and I were tested, I imagined if we were both positive, even though our decisions might have been different, whatever route we took, we would take together. When I tested negative, after the initial tears of joy and the feeling of dodging the bullet, I wondered why my sister wasn't negative too. Why must she go through the unthinkable while I carry on with my life? It didn't seem fair. I remember thinking that for once, God seemed to be on our side, as I have two daughters and my sister has no children. If nothing else, this could be the end of the BRCA mutation in our family. Whenever I felt guilty about being negative, I used that thought as a way to feel better. Looking back, I don't think I would have had my sister's strength and courage. Given a choice, she too would have been negative, but if someone in our family had to be positive, she would have wanted it to be her. —LINDA

THE FORCE PERSPECTIVE: TAKING TIME TO PROCESS, GRIEVE, AND ADJUST

Our interactions with thousands of women who have had genetic testing for a BRCA mutation reveal a wide range of emotions:

- fear, anxiety, or sadness knowing they have a mutation
- loss of innocence or safety

- surprise at their reaction to positive results (for example, if they've had cancer and underestimated how a positive result might make them feel)
- pressure (from themselves or loved ones) and frustration because they feel scared or sad instead of grateful for not having cancer
- grateful for the knowledge genetic testing provides
- relieved to finally understand why they or their loved ones developed cancer
- guilt about possibly passing a mutation to their children
- relieved to have tested negative
- guilt for testing negative, particularly when a close relative tests positive
- concern about stopping intense cancer surveillance, even when a test is a true negative
- anger, frustration, or sadness because of ambiguous test results and how they make risk management decisions more difficult

Learning you have a mutation is big news. Even if you think you're prepared for it, sometimes the reality is more traumatic than you expected. And that's okay. There's no right or wrong way to feel. You can learn to accept your results, but it may take time to process the implications and work through your feelings. Remind loved ones to allow you that time as well. Talking with a mental health professional, clergy, trusted friend, relative, or counselor can help you sort out your feelings and make decisions about your risk.

WHAT TO REMEMBER ABOUT GENETIC TEST RESULTS

- Genetic tests identify known mutations. Other undiscovered mutations may also affect cancer risk.
- Testing positive doesn't guarantee you'll develop cancer. Testing negative doesn't guarantee that you won't.
- Most people don't need to make decisions right away. Take time to process your feelings and adjust to the information.
- A genetic counselor can help you understand your test result and how it affects your risk.

LEARN MORE ABOUT GENETIC TEST RESULTS

Your genetic counselor is always the best resource for understanding test results.

The Negative BRCA Test website (www.negativebrcatest.com) will help you understand your negative test result and potential next steps.

Positive Results, by Joi L. Morris and Ora K. Gordon, M.D., is a memoir and guidebook for women at high risk for breast and ovarian cancer.

PART THREE MANAGING YOUR RISK

Your DNA Doesn't Have to Be Your Destiny

Chapter 8 **Early Detection**

Strategies

THE NEXT BEST THING TO PREVENTING CANCER is catching it early, when it's more likely to be cured. That's why surveillance is so important. It doesn't prevent cancer or reduce risk, but if a tumor develops, surveillance offers the opportunity to find it before it spreads.

High-Risk Surveillance for Breast Cancer

Routine cancer screenings recommended for the general population aren't adequate for high-risk women, who

- tend to develop breast cancer when younger, before routine screening in the general population begins.
- need screening beginning at a younger age, when breasts are more dense and mammography is less effective.
- have a higher lifetime risk for cancer.

If you have an elevated risk for breast cancer and still have your natural breasts, your screening repertoire should include all the actions listed in table 7.

The Vocabulary of Screening

Scientists use certain criteria to describe the utility of screening tests. *Sensitivity* is the probability of a true positive test among those who have the disease—if two women in a group of one hundred have cancer, a highly sensitive test would correctly identify both. A highly sensitive

Table 7. NCCN guidelines for breast cancer surveillance

Screening method	Average risk	BRCA mutation
Breast self-exam	Education about optional BSE at age 20	BSE training starting at age 18
Clinical breast exam	Every 3 years during 20s and 30s, and annually, starting at age 40	Every 6–12 months, starting at age 25
Mammogram	Annually, starting at age 40	Annually, starting at age 25 or 5–10 years before earliest age of onset in family
MRI	Not recommended	Annually, starting at age 25 or 5–10 years before earliest age of onset in family

Note: If you're at high risk (lifetime risk of 20 percent or higher) for breast cancer and don't have a BRCA mutation, the American Cancer Society recommends annual breast MRI in addition to mammography.

test doesn't miss many cancers, though it's more likely to identify normal tissue as suspicious (false-positive), leading to more unnecessary biopsies. *Specificity* is the probability of a true negative test among those who don't have the disease. A highly specific test correctly identifies normal tissue—if only two women in the group of one hundred have cancer, yet ten falsely test positive, the test isn't very specific. A highly specific test is less likely to produce false positives, but it may also miss more cancers. The ideal test is both sensitive and specific—if someone tests positive, they have the disease. If they test negative, they don't. It's difficult, if not impossible, to develop the ideal test, and screening methods usually compromise one quality or the other.

Breast Exams

You and a healthcare professional should carefully examine your breasts for changes and abnormalities. Performing routine breast self-

exams (BSE) has long been recommended. It may cause false positives—
women who practice regular BSE have more biopsies for benign lumps
than women who don't. Many women, particularly those at high risk, discover their own early stage breast tumors during BSE or while dressing,
showering, or bathing. A Harvard study found that 71 percent of women
diagnosed with breast cancer at age 40 or younger discovered their breast
cancers by self-exam.[1] Duke University researchers demonstrated that
BSE can detect new breast cancers in high-risk women: "Our results provide evidence that BSE should not be abandoned as an adjunct for breast
cancer education, as well as a surveillance tool for high-risk women."[2]

Self-exams need to be done regularly and done well. It's a good idea
to have a healthcare professional show you how to do a BSE and review
your technique to make sure you're doing it correctly. The Susan G.
Komen for the Cure website (www.komen.org) has a good instructional
video. Become familiar with the landscape of your breasts, both on the
surface and the underlying tissue, so you'll know if something feels or
looks different. Examine your breasts at the same time each month a
few days after your period or, if you're postmenopausal, on the same day
each month.

A clinical breast exam (CBE) is performed by your primary doctor (usually during your annual physical), a gynecologist, or another
healthcare professional. You might wonder why you should bother with
monthly BSE if a doctor is going to examine your breasts anyway. While
a CBE is an important part of your screening regimen—it's an opportunity for an expert to detect any suspicious breast changes—it only occurs
twice a year. You, on the other hand, have twelve opportunities in the
same period to find anything unusual. Used alone, CBE is a somewhat
ineffective method of finding breast cancer. Combining self-exams,
mammography, and MRI improves the odds of finding early tumors.

Mammograms

Overall, mammography is an effective tool for identifying early stage
breast cancer. Mammograms use low-dose x-rays to produce images

of the internal breast structure, often finding *microcalcifications*, tiny calcium deposits that may precede a tumor long before it can be felt. Mammography isn't a perfect technology. It misses some breast cancers (false negatives), especially in younger women with dense breasts, and it isn't highly sensitive. It frequently identifies suspicious changes that create anxiety, require biopsies, and turn out to be noncancerous (false positives). If you're unfamiliar with mammograms, you'll find a helpful video at www.mayoclinic.com (search for "mammogram video").

MY STORY: Mammography Saved My Life

A mammogram found my breast cancer at age 40. My tumor was just 1.7 cm and couldn't be felt by me or my surgeon. Without that mammogram, my cancer would have gone undetected. More than likely, it would have spread to my lymph nodes and who knows where else.   —SHAWN

If you've ever taken photographs with film then upgraded to a digital camera, you can appreciate the difference between traditional and digital mammography, a newer technology that produces instant, sharper computerized images that can be enlarged to more easily spot breast abnormalities. It's more sensitive than standard mammography, so fewer women need to repeat the process. It's also safe. Digital mammography emits up to 50 percent less radiation, although the amount in newer film mammography is also quite small. In a large clinical trial sponsored by the National Cancer Institute, both technologies performed equally well among 50,000 U.S. and Canadian women who showed no signs of breast cancer. Digital mammography was significantly better at screening women who were under age 50, who were of any age with very dense breasts, or who were premenopausal or perimenopausal at any age (women who had a last menstrual period within twelve months of their mammograms).[3] Some of the 10,000 U.S. facilities that now use conventional mammography are converting to digital technology, but it will be some time before it's widely available.

Mammograms for Women under Age 30

Being at high risk means you're more likely to develop breast cancer at a younger age than other women, so it makes sense to begin having mammograms sooner. How early is too early? NCCN high-risk guidelines suggest starting at age 25 or five to ten years before the earliest onset in your family. Some experts propose that the increased lifetime exposure to radiation from starting annual mammograms before age 30 could lead to slightly increased breast cancer risk. It's unclear to what extent risk is increased, and little long-term research is available on the effects of radiation in BRCA mutation carriers. When researchers addressed this issue with mathematical computer models, they calculated that for every 10,000 women between ages 25 and 30, early mammograms would save twelve or fewer lives, while the radiation received might cause about fifty-one breast cancer deaths ten or more years later. The effect was reversed among BRCA carriers age 30 and older: mammograms were estimated to save more lives than would be lost to radiation-induced breast cancers.[4] More research is needed to better determine the benefits and risks of mammography in young women with mutations.

Mammograms for Women over Age 65

One revealing study comparing ten years of Medicare data showed that women are less likely to have mammograms as they get older.[5] Study authors surmised that doctors less frequently recommend routine mammograms for older women, who often seek health care for specific problems, rather than for prevention. Even though much of a previvor's cancer risk occurs before age 50, it persists throughout life. So it's important to remain vigilant and continue having routine mammograms—they're particularly good at identifying older women's breast cancers—especially if you're at high risk.

Mammograms after Breast Cancer

If you had breast cancer that was treated with radiation or chemotherapy, your doctor will probably recommend a new baseline mammogram six months after your final treatment, then annually thereafter. Some doctors recommend mammograms at six-month intervals for two or three years following radiation. If you've had one breast removed, you need annual mammograms of your healthy breast to address your increased risk of developing another breast cancer. Experience counts! Check the U.S. Food and Drug Administration mammography facility database (www.accessdata.fda.gov /scripts/cdrh/cfdocs/cfMQSA/mqsa.cfm) to verify that your mammogram facility is FDA certified. Most doctors don't recommend mammograms after bilateral mastectomy, whether or not your breasts are reconstructed, because almost all of your breast tissue is gone.

> **MAMMOGRAPHY SCREENINGS WHEN YOU HAVE IMPLANTS**
>
> If your natural breasts have been enlarged with implants, your mammograms should be performed by specially trained technicians. Ask your doctor for a referral, or inquire about a facility's experience when you make your appointment. Always let the radiology technician know before your screening that you have implants. The FDA recommends MRI to check for ruptures at three years after placement of silicone implants for augmentation or reconstruction, and every two years thereafter.

Magnetic Resonance Imaging (MRI)

MRI uses magnetic fields and radio waves instead of radiation to produce hundreds of detailed images of the breast from several angles. Specially designed breast MRI machines produce the best images (some facilities don't have them). Breast MRI is different than MRIs used to scan the head or chest and may be particularly good at finding cancers missed by mammograms, especially in premenopausal women. MRI is sensitive, so it's also particularly good at finding abnormalities, including those that prove to be benign, which means it's less specific than other breast cancer tests. Even though a biopsy is required to prove that an abnormality is benign, experts believe the benefit of MRI outweighs the downside for high-risk women. When an MRI detects an abnormality that can't be seen by mammography or ultrasound, a special MRI-guided biopsy is required. Traditional biopsy methods aren't effective, yet not all facilities that offer breast MRI have MRI-guided biopsy. Before you make an appointment, ask how many breast-screening MRIs a facility has performed, what their biopsy recommendation rate is, and whether they can perform MRI-guided biopsies if your screening finds something suspicious.

According to the American Cancer Society, you're considered high risk if your lifetime odds of developing breast cancer are estimated to be 20 percent or greater. It's an important distinction, because it means you should have breast MRIs in addition to the routine mammograms suggested for women of average risk. Having a BRCA mutation, a family history of breast cancer, or another hereditary syndrome meets the high-risk criteria.

Comparing MRI and Mammography

Most studies find MRI to be more sensitive, yet used together, mammograms and MRI are complementary, with each finding some cancers missed by the other. According to research, adding MRI to mammography improves sensitivity from 40 to 94 percent for finding cancer in young high-risk women.[6] MRI is also good at finding early cancers in premenopausal, high-risk women whose younger, dense breast tissue can obscure mammography images. If MRI finds more tumors in high-risk women, why isn't it the hands-down screening technology of choice? Mammograms have a distinct advantage: they pick up more microcalcifications that may be DCIS. Although imperfect and less sensitive, they're more widely available, less expensive, and produce fewer false positives.

The Future of Breast Cancer Screening?

Digital tomosynthesis uses x-rays to create computerized three-dimensional pictures of the breast. A woman is positioned as though she will have a mammogram, and an x-ray tube quickly takes pictures from different angles as it moves around her breast. Scientists hope digital tomosynthesis will eliminate the sensitivity and specificity shortcomings of mammograms and MRIs. Two other experimental techniques are also promising. *Molecular breast imaging,* or breast-specific gamma imaging, uses a radioactive tracer injected into a vein to highlight any cancerous areas in the breast. Another procedure, *positron emission mammography,* detects even very small lesions by tracking sugar as it's metabolized by tumors. Both processes may reduce the need for redoing images and lower the biopsy rates associated with MRI. Unlike MRI, both involve exposure to radiation. All three procedures are currently limited to research.

High-Risk Surveillance for Ovarian Cancer

We have no self-exam or "mammogram" to find early stage ovarian tumors, and contrary to common belief, Pap smears don't screen for this disease. Because no current test reliably detects ovarian cancer, no screening guidelines exist for symptomless women in the general population, where the risk of ovarian cancer is low. NCCN guidelines for high-risk women include those listed in table 8.

Table 8. NCCN guidelines for ovarian cancer surveillance

Screening method	*Women of average risk*	*Women with a BRCA mutation*
Pelvic exam*	Annually to assess reproductive organs; doesn't screen for ovarian cancer	Every 6–12 months, starting at age 30–35 or 5–10 years before the earliest age of onset in family
Transvaginal ultrasound with color Doppler*	Not recommended	Same frequency as pelvic exam
CA-125 blood test*	Not recommended	Same frequency as pelvic exam

*preferably on day 1–10 of the menstrual cycle for premenopausal women

Pelvic Exam

A pelvic exam checks for abnormalities of the reproductive system. It should include a rectovaginal exam: the healthcare provider feels the ovaries by inserting a gloved, lubricated finger into the rectum and another finger into the vagina at the same time using the other hand to press on the abdomen. As uncomfortable as it may sound, the exam shouldn't be painful. It's the best way to feel the position, size, and shape of the ovaries. A pelvic exam might pick up an abnormality that could indicate cancer, even though it's not sensitive or specific enough to identify ovarian cancer with certainty. Nevertheless, it should be part of a thorough exam for all adult women, no matter what their risk.

Transvaginal Ultrasound with Color Doppler

Transvaginal ultrasound uses a small probe inserted into the vagina to look for abnormalities of the ovaries, tubes, and uterus. A large study of ultrasound screening in high-risk women showed that most ovarian cancers were diagnosed at stage 3 or higher. All the women had normal scans during the previous year, leading researchers to conclude that ultrasound doesn't dependably identify early stage ovarian cancer.[7] Retrospective research of ovarian cancer that was detected by screening concluded that *high-grade serous* ovarian tumors (the type that usually develops in BRCA carriers) are more likely to be diagnosed only after they have advanced. Even though transvaginal ultrasound isn't highly sensitive or specific and can lead to unnecessary surgery, experts recommend it for high-risk women who still have their ovaries.

CA-125 Blood Test

CA-125 is a blood protein that is sometimes elevated when a woman has ovarian cancer. After a diagnosis, a CA-125 test is used to monitor response to treatment. Once treatment is completed, the test helps to determine whether the cancer has returned. As a method of routine screening, CA-125 produces less than optimal results in most women: about 50 percent of women with early stage ovarian cancer and 20 percent who have advanced disease don't have elevated CA-125 levels.[8] Liver disease, uterine fibroids, other benign conditions, or other cancers can also raise CA-125 levels, especially in premenopausal women, making the test difficult to interpret, producing false positives, and requiring surgery to confirm a diagnosis. Undependable for most women, CA-125 combined with transvaginal ultrasound may find some ovarian cancers before symptoms appear and is recommended for high-risk women. Researchers are trying to determine whether measuring CA-125 levels every three months in high-risk women improves the test's sensitivity and specificity.

Biomarkers for Early Detection of Ovarian Cancer

We've mapped the human genome and identified many disease-causing gene mutations. The next step in our quest for early detection is searching for other *biomarkers,* biological indicators of disease. Figuring out which biomarkers signal different cancers and developing a test to measure them would improve surveillance of early stage tumors. Sounds easy. It isn't. CA-125 is a good example. We know it's a biomarker for ovarian cancer, yet the current test doesn't accurately determine who has the disease and who doesn't. Combining CA-125 tests with other biomarkers could improve both the sensitivity and specificity of detecting ovarian cancer. The false-positive concern—needing surgery to follow up on a suspicious test result that may prove false—remains a large hurdle. New discoveries are bringing us closer to the answers we need to develop a dependable surveillance method for ovarian cancer.

What should sensitivity and specificity standards be for previvors, who have a higher prevalence of ovarian cancer than the general population? The answer may depend on your age, personal circumstances, and tolerance for potential false positives. If you're already considering prophylactic *salpingo-oophorectomy* (removal of your ovaries), you may be willing to trade specificity for increased sensitivity; you might worry more about missing an existing ovarian cancer than receiving a false-positive result. We desperately need a dependable way to find early stage ovarian cancer. In medicine, there's always a need to strike a balance between making something available because we need it now and ensuring it stands up to the rigors of good scientific research. Researchers continue to work to identify tests that can accurately detect early stage ovarian cancer.

EXPERT VIEW: The Challenge of Early Stage Ovarian Cancer Screening

BY NOAH D. KAUFF, M.D.

Ovarian cancer is rare, even in women with inherited risk. Much of the early detection research for this disease has focused on comparing blood samples to isolate proteins or other chemicals that may distinguish women with ovarian cancer compared to healthy women. These studies have discovered biomarkers that have the potential to indicate the presence of ovarian cancer; the greater challenge is finding markers that reliably indicate the disease in its early stages.

Since most ovarian cancer is diagnosed when advanced, studies rarely have the opportunity to include enough women with early stage disease. To improve patient outcomes, we need to identify biomarkers that signal ovarian cancer in stage 1, when it is still confined to the ovary or fallopian tube. The next step would be validation of the test: can it detect early cancer in healthy, high-risk women and not mistakenly identify women who do not have the disease? The consequence of a screening test missing an ovarian cancer can mean lower likelihood of survival. Conversely, the consequence of a test that is not specific can be the fear and anxiety caused by a false-positive test, as well as the risks of an invasive exploratory surgery to determine if cancer is present. Our goal is to find a test with near-perfect sensitivity and specificity so that the benefits of ovarian cancer screening outweigh the risks. In the meantime, salpingo-oophorectomy is very effective in reducing risk and remains the standard of care for women with mutations in BRCA1 or BRCA2 after childbearing is complete.

MY STORY: Depending on Surveillance . . . for Now

I plan to wait until I'm 40 to have prophylactic oophorectomy. While I have a BRCA2 mutation, my family has no known cases of ovarian cancer. I'm not ready to abandon the desire to have a biological child, and I want to keep my body working as well as it can with my own hormones, for as long as I can. I feel confident that I can use increased surveillance to keep my ovaries as long as it's safe for me to do so.   —BETHANN

Is It Cancer?

If screening procedures identify abnormal or questionable tissue changes in the breasts or ovaries, a biopsy is usually required to verify whether the change is benign or malignant.

Breast Biopsies

Examining cells under a microscope is the usual method of identifying cancer; to do that, your physician must first withdraw sample cells. If you have a lump that can be felt, your surgeon may recommend a *fine needle aspiration* to remove cells or a surgical biopsy to remove a piece of tissue. Aspiration involves inserting an ultra-thin hollow needle and removing cells or fluid. This is the easiest and least invasive way to determine if the lump is a fluid-filled cyst or a solid mass that should be further evaluated. Unfortunately, needle samples don't always yield enough cells, and cells are sometimes damaged during aspiration.

Your doctor may perform a *core needle biopsy* instead, inserting a somewhat larger hollow tube into the breast to remove a more generous sample. Other than a slight sting from local anesthesia, needle biopsies are often painless, don't take much time, and don't typically leave scars. You head home soon after with just a small bandage and slight bruising and may need nothing more than an ice pack and over-the-counter pain medication.

If your lump is too small to be felt, your doctor may recommend a mammogram, MRI, or ultrasound to help guide the surgeon or radiologist to its exact location. Breast ultrasound bounces high-frequency sound waves off tissue to produce a *sonogram*, the same technology that creates computerized images of a fetus during pregnancy. Ultrasound doesn't detect microcalcifications as effectively as mammography, and it isn't routinely used to screen for breast cancer. It's sometimes used to better view abnormalities found by other screening procedures. Ultrasound distinguishes fluid-filled cysts from solid masses, so it's often used to evaluate lumps not easily seen by mammography.

Stereotactic biopsies use images of your breast taken by a digital mammogram or ultrasound. A computer-guided needle locates the exact site of the abnormality; then a surgeon makes a tiny incision (about ¼" long) and removes several cell samples with a syringe or a special vacuum-powered probe.

A surgical biopsy is the most conclusive way to determine whether an abnormality is cancer. It may be necessary if you have very small breasts; if the suspicious area is close to the chest wall, the nipple, or the surface of the breast; if a needle biopsy is inconclusive; or if the questionable area is too large to be sampled by needle. Your surgeon may perform an incisional biopsy, removing only a portion of the lump, or an excisional biopsy to remove it entirely. Removing the entire lump is more effective if it's small, because it presents less possibility for false negatives. When a biopsy sample includes cancerous tissue, the surgeon removes any additional malignant tissue around the tumor until the surrounding margins are clear of cancerous cells. After the biopsy, if a pathologist finds that the margins of the tissue sample still contain cancer cells, the surgeon may need to re-operate to remove additional tissue until no signs of cancer remain. This is referred to as obtaining *clear* or *clean margins.* Surgical biopsies are outpatient procedures involving minimal swelling and bruising, and small incisions that scar. Any discomfort is usually managed by pain medication. Sometimes surgeons leave a small metal marker or clip that helps them to identify the area on later MRI screenings or mammogram.

Ovarian Surgery

Surgery is the only conclusive way to determine whether a suspicious pelvic mass is cancerous. If cancer is found, outcomes are better when surgery is performed by a gynecologic oncologist.[9] An OB-GYN may only sample the ovaries; gynecologic oncologists are trained to identify ovarian cancer, assess its severity, stage it, and aggressively remove any cancer that has spread beyond the original tumor. The FDA-approved OVA1 blood test checks CA-125 and four other proteins that are either increased or reduced when ovarian cancer is present. It can indicate whether a pelvic mass is likely to be benign or malignant prior to exploratory surgery. An abnormal result indicates a higher likelihood of cancer; the next step is referral to a gynecologic oncologist for follow-up.

Screening for Other Hereditary Cancers
Colorectal Cancer

If you have Lynch syndrome, you're at high risk for colon cancer, a disease that begins with benign polyps or growths. You need routine colonoscopies to find and remove any colorectal tumors as early as possible. Performed under mild anesthesia, the painless procedure involves placing a flexible scope into the rectum, examining the entire colon, and removing any polyps. Virtual colonoscopy uses computed tomography (CT), a type of computerized x-ray, to closely examine the colon, so it involves some exposure to radiation and may not be covered by insurance.

Fallopian Tube and Primary Peritoneal Cancer

Women at high risk for ovarian cancer also have increased risk for fallopian tube and primary peritoneal cancer, although these cancers develop rarely. Fallopian tube cancer is most often discovered during prophylactic surgery to remove the ovaries. Screening for these cancers unfortunately depends on the same methods currently used for ovarian cancer: CA-125, pelvic exam, and transvaginal ultrasound. (A promising new scoping procedure is described in chapter 12.) Transvaginal ultrasound and CA-125 are usually not required after your ovaries and tubes are removed.

Pancreatic Cancer

We currently have no way to screen for pancreatic cancer; 75 percent of diagnoses are advanced when discovered. This disease is rare, even in people with hereditary cancer risk, and surgery is required to determine whether a suspicious area is harmless or cancerous. Researchers are trying to develop a blood test that can accurately screen for pancreatic cancer and are exploring whether *endoscopic ultrasound*—passing a tiny scope with an ultrasound probe down the esophagus to the stomach—can effectively examine the pancreas, find abnormalities, and hopefully detect early stage cancer in people at high risk for this disease.

Stomach and Esophageal Cancer

Screening tests for stomach and esophageal cancers are similar and are recommended only for people who have elevated risk for these cancers. Under anesthesia, doctors insert a thin flexible scope through the esophagus and stomach to check for abnormalities. Your level of risk for these cancers determines when you should start screening and how frequently screening procedures should be performed.

Uterine (Endometrial) Cancer

The American Cancer Society recommends informing women about the risks and symptoms of uterine cancer as they enter menopause. Immediately advise your doctor of any unexpected vaginal bleeding or spotting. If you have Lynch syndrome or other factors that put you at high risk, talk to your doctor about transvaginal ultrasound or endometrial biopsy beginning at age 35.

Melanoma

Existing screening guidelines for melanoma advise yearly exams by a dermatologist who has expertise in diagnosing skin cancer but address only the general population. The exam includes checking your skin from head to toe for any suspicious moles or skin changes. You should also routinely do this yourself. Become familiar with your skin so you'll notice any new moles or unusual changes—notify your doctor if you do. If you have a BRCA2 mutation, you should probably also have an annual eye exam by an ophthalmologist, including pupil dilation and examination of the retina, because some forms of melanoma affect the eyes. Talk with your oncologist and eye doctor about when you should begin these screenings and how often you should have them.

Prostate Cancer

Men with BRCA mutations need annual screening for prostate cancer (discussed in chapter 17).

INSURANCE AND PAYMENT ISSUES

Medicare, Medicaid, and most health insurance plans cover all routine annual screenings, including mammogram. The Patient Protection and Affordable Care Act requires health plans issued after September 23, 2010 to cover the full cost, without copays or deductibles, of annual in-network screening mammograms for women age 40 and older, and routine colonoscopies. The requirement doesn't extend to plans established before that date. (Visit www.healthreform.gov for more details.)

Some insurers now consider MRI screening as medically necessary for high-risk individuals and pay for one annual MRI test if ordered by your doctor; you may need a letter from your doctor to cover tests beginning at age 25. If you don't have insurance or can't pay for standard-of-care surveillance, ask your doctor or contact your local hospital or American

Cancer Society office. The National Breast and Cervical Cancer Early Detection Program (www.cdc.gov/cancer/nbccedp) provides free mammograms and breast exams (and Pap tests) for low-income, uninsured, and underserved women.

WHAT TO REMEMBER ABOUT EARLY DETECTION

- Early detection strategies try to catch cancer early (not prevent it), when it's most treatable.
- High-risk women need to begin surveillance at a younger age than other women.
- Current guidelines recommend both mammograms and MRIs for high-risk women.
- Current ovarian cancer screening methods don't usually identify early stage tumors.

LEARN MORE ABOUT EARLY DETECTION

National Comprehensive Cancer Network (www.nccn.org) guidelines dictate the standard of care for cancer surveillance in high-risk patients and are updated annually.

The Imaginis website has information about mammography (www.imaginis.com/mammogram/directory-of-mammography-articles) and MRI breast imaging (www.imaginis.com/breast-health/magnetic-resonance-breast-imaging-mri-mr-3).

Clinical trials are important opportunities to participate in new screening technologies and procedures. See the clinical trials registry at clinicaltrials.gov.

Chapter 9 Chemoprevention

IF YOU'RE CONSIDERING OPTIONS to reduce your cancer risk, you have two choices: chemoprevention, as described in this chapter, and surgery (chapters 10 and 12). Taking chemoprevention medications doesn't guarantee you'll never develop cancer, but it can decrease your risk. If you still have your breasts and ovaries, you'll need to maintain surveillance to find any early cancers. Some women take chemoprevention drugs and then later further reduce their risk with surgery.

Chemoprevention isn't for everyone. You may welcome its noninvasive risk-reducing potential or may decide the possible side effects outweigh the benefits, depending on your overall health and tolerance for risk. Some studies of these medications haven't specifically focused on high-risk women; fewer have focused specifically on BRCA mutation carriers. A healthcare team with expertise in managing high-risk patients can give you a clear sense of how various chemoprevention drugs might affect your risk.

Risk-Reducing Medications for Breast Cancer

Tamoxifen and raloxifene are FDA-approved medications that reduce the risk of developing breast cancer in high-risk women. Both are *selective estrogen receptor modulators* (SERMs), drugs that block estrogen. Another SERM, fareston, is used to treat postmenopausal metastatic breast cancer. It isn't approved for chemoprevention.

Tamoxifen

Well-studied tamoxifen (marketed as Nolvadex tablets and Soltamox liquid) has been standard treatment for ER+ breast cancers since 1977. The drug has an impressive track record for treating breast cancer and lowering recurrence. Study data show tamoxifen:

- shrinks large ER+ tumors before surgery.
- cuts in half the risk of a new cancer in the opposite breast.
- lowers recurrence 40 to 50 percent in postmenopausal women and 30 to 50 percent in premenopausal women.
- reduces risk of recurring DCIS or invasive breast cancer by 50 percent when used after lumpectomy and radiation treatment for DCIS.

Researchers have studied the benefit of tamoxifen in different populations of women, with different results for each group. In a study of women with BRCA-related cancer in one breast, those who took tamoxifen demonstrated a significantly reduced risk in the other breast.[1] The medication appeared to work for both BRCA1 and BRCA2 mutation carriers. The research on tamoxifen for previvors shows different results. A large U.S. study showed that tamoxifen substantially reduced the chance for breast cancer in high-risk women.[2] Most participants didn't have BRCA mutations. Among the nineteen women with BRCA mutations, only those with a mutation in BRCA2 benefited. The medication didn't seem to help women who had BRCA1 mutations. A second study in the United Kingdom reviewed a similar group of high-risk women who took tamoxifen for eight years and were then followed for twenty years.[3] Participants weren't tested to determine whether any of them had BRCA mutations. This study showed a reduced risk for ER+ breast cancers, but not for ER− breast cancers.

Based on this limited research, most experts believe tamoxifen effectively decreases risk for breast cancer in survivors and previvors, especially those who have BRCA2 mutations. Not all experts agree that it is equally effective for BRCA1 mutation carriers, who tend to develop

ER– cancers. If you're considering tamoxifen for chemoprevention, discuss the benefits and limitations with your oncologist.

Raloxifene

Marketed as Evista, raloxifene functions much like tamoxifen, with less risk for uterine cancers. Raloxifene was originally developed to prevent and treat osteoporosis, but doctors noticed that women who took it for bone loss had a reduced risk of invasive breast cancer. The Study of Tamoxifen and Raloxifene (STAR) trial in 1999 showed that both medications reduced high-risk postmenopausal women's odds (as defined by the Gail Model) of developing invasive breast cancer by about half during the five years they took it and for ten years following. Based on these results, raloxifene is FDA approved for breast cancer prevention in postmenopausal women. No studies have yet explored whether it prevents breast cancer specifically in BRCA mutation carriers. Raloxifene also works against DCIS, which can develop into breast cancer, and LCIS. Compared to tamoxifen, the benefits of raloxifene decline more quickly once women stop taking it.

Side Effects of SERMs

Tamoxifen and raloxifene are reliable and effective multitasking medications.

SOME ANTIDEPRESSANTS MAY REDUCE TAMOXIFEN'S EFFECTIVENESS

Drugs often interact with other drugs, and some evidence shows that specific antidepressants in the group of drugs known as *serotonin specific reuptake inhibitors* (SSRIs) may affect tamoxifen metabolism in the body, making it less effective. Many breast cancer patients take these SSRIs to manage hot flashes or depression caused by hormonal treatment. If you decide to take tamoxifen and you already take Paxil, Prozac, Wellbutrin, or another antidepressant, discuss it with your doctor, who may consider an alternative such as Celexa, Effexor, or Lexapro. Your doctor can also determine if any of your other medicines, vitamins, or supplements should be reconsidered. If you currently take tamoxifen, don't abruptly quit your antidepressant. Your doctor can help decide whether any change in medication is warranted and, if so, the best way to wean away from one drug or switch to a substitute.

Aside from potentially preventing breast cancer, they improve bone density. Both, however, have side effects. Taking either medication may cause hot flashes, vaginal dryness, mood changes, and other menopause-like symptoms, which may be mild and well tolerated by some women; others need medication to address their symptoms. SERMs can also cause vaginal bleeding or discharge, headaches, nausea, leg cramps, rashes, and other serious side effects.

Tamoxifen slightly increases a woman's risk for endometrial cancer—the risk is still relatively low, about two chances in 1,000 per year.[4] Raloxifene has less risk of uterine cancer. Unlike tamoxifen, it doesn't have an estrogen-like effect on the uterus. These medications also increase the chance of stroke and blood clots, particularly in those who smoke or have clotting disorders. Neither drug is appropriate for women with a Factor V Leiden mutation, those who have (or have had) blood clots, or those taking estrogen replacement or certain cholesterol-reducing drugs, including Locholest and Questran.

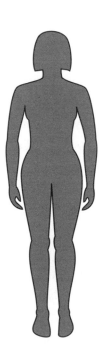

Effects of Tamoxifen

Good effects

- Reduces risk of ER+ breast cancer
- More effective against invasive breast cancer
- Benefits persist when it's no longer taken
- Strengthens bones
- Lowers LDL cholesterol

Bad effects

- Increases risk of uterine cancer
- Increases risk of blood clots
- Causes menopause-like symptoms

Effects of Raloxifene

Good effects

- More effective against noninvasive breast cancer
- Strengthens bones
- Lowers LDL cholesterol
- Less risk for uterine cancer than with tamoxifen

Bad effects

- Benefits decline when it's no longer taken
- Increases risk for blood clots, but less than with tamoxifen
- Causes menopause-like symptoms, but fewer than with tamoxifen

Comparing tamoxifen and raloxifene

Aromatase Inhibitors

Aromatase inhibitors (AIs), including exemestane (Aromasin), letro-zole (Femara), and anastrozole (Arimidex) treat postmenopausal ER+ and PR+ breast cancers. For survivors, AIs work more effectively than tamoxifen against advanced breast cancer; following five years of tamox-ifen with five years of an AI continues to reduce your risk of recurrence. Health experts are hoping AIs prevent breast cancer in postmenopausal previvors as successfully as they treat breast cancers in women with spo-radic, hormone-positive breast cancers.

You may wonder why postmenopausal women need to be concerned about estrogen. After menopause, even though your ovaries don't pro-duce much estrogen, your body converts fat and other hormones into estrogen to a lesser degree than before menopause; it's still enough to stimulate estrogen receptors on the breast. This is one reason why being overweight contributes to breast cancer risk. While tamoxifen and ral-oxifene block estrogen from breast cancer receptors, AIs reduce up to 95 percent of postmenopausal estrogen. AIs don't affect the amount of estrogen made by the ovaries; that's why they're not effective for pre-menopausal women. Unlike SERMs, AIs don't improve bone density. In fact, they may accelerate postmenopausal bone loss. Unlike tamox-ifen and raloxifene, AIs are less likely to cause serious blood clots and don't cause uterine cancers—they can cause hot flashes, vaginal dry-ness, headaches, muscle or joint pain, and other short-term side effects similar to those caused by tamoxifen.

AIs aren't FDA approved to prevent breast cancer. They could be prescribed as a preventive measure in the future if research shows they effectively reduce risk. AIs haven't been studied as much as SERMs, so experts don't yet know about their long-term effects or risks. The Arimi-dex, Tamoxifen, Alone or in Combination (ATAC) trial found Arimidex reduced the risk of a new cancer in the opposite breast of survivors by 58 percent.[5] The study didn't specifically include women with BRCA mutations, so its preventive benefits in mutation carriers remains uncer-tain. Clinical studies are under way to determine whether AIs reduce postmenopausal breast cancer in high-risk women, including BRCA carriers. You can track the status of these trials at clinicaltrials.gov.

MY STORY: For Me, Surveillance Alone Isn't Enough

When I tested positive for a BRCA1 mutation at age 27, I wasn't ready for prophylactic surgery to reduce my risk, so my oncologist suggested I take tamoxifen for five years. I knew it was controversial for prevention, but I researched it carefully. If my body didn't react well to surgical menopause or I had complications from mastectomy, that could affect my life forever. Taking a pill didn't feel that way, and I would be doing something more than just surveillance. I decided to try it for six months; if I didn't like how I felt or couldn't handle the side effects, I would stop taking it. I was comfortable with my decision, and I had an easy out if I didn't want to continue. As it turned out, I tolerated tamoxifen very well, maybe because I was so young when I started taking it or because I was proactive with my diet and lifestyle. Maybe I was just lucky. I took a risk with tamoxifen; it was the best decision I could have made. —CARI

Alternatives under Study
Nonsteroidal Anti-inflammatory Drugs

Because inflammation contributes to many diseases, including cancers, some scientists speculate that aspirin and other anti-inflammatory medications might reduce cancer risk. Research to analyze the effects of aspirin and other nonsteroidal anti-inflammatory drugs (NSAIDs) on breast cancer risk has been inconclusive, and studies haven't specifically focused on high-risk individuals. NSAIDs include several common over-the-counter painkillers, including ibuprofen (Advil, Motrin, and others) and naproxen sodium (Aleve).

In the Women's Health Initiative, a national fifteen-year study of cardiovascular disease, cancer, and osteoporosis in postmenopausal women, individuals over age 50 who used aspirin regularly had a 21 percent decreased chance of developing breast cancer.[6] Regular use of ibuprofen was associated with a 49 percent reduction in breast cancer risk, even in women who had first-degree female relatives (mother, sister, or daughter) with breast cancer. The study was observational only: women who regularly took NSAIDs were less likely to develop breast cancer, but researchers can't be certain if the NSAIDs or some other factor produced the benefit. Nor did the study specifically focus on high-risk women. The Nurses' Health Study, a large, long-term research effort following 76,821 nurses, showed that aspirin or other NSAIDs taken at least twice weekly don't reduce premenopausal breast cancer risk.[7]

Certain NSAIDs increase the potential for death from heart disease. A clinical trial studying whether Celebrex could lessen the risk for colon polyps was discontinued when participants who took the medication suffered more heart disease and related deaths compared to participants who took a placebo. Even though the risk of heart disease-related death was low—about 3 percent of people taking the highest dose and 2 percent risk in those who were taking a lower dose—in this particular study, the risks of Celebrex outweighed the benefits.[8] Other clinical trials are exploring whether nonsteroidal anti-inflammatory agents decrease breast cancer in high-risk women, including some studies of BRCA mutation carriers. Some medications in this category, including Celebrex and others, increase the risk of heart attack and stroke and shouldn't be used by anyone at high risk for those conditions.

Fenretinide

Research suggests that fenretinide, a medication related to vitamin A, might prevent new breast tumors in premenopausal women who have been previously diagnosed. Over fifteen years, 1,739 patients previously diagnosed with DCIS or stage 1 breast cancer who weren't treated with chemotherapy took fenretinide and had 17 percent lower incidence of a second breast cancer diagnosis than women who didn't take the medication. Fenretinide was effective primarily in premenopausal women; the younger the woman, the more fenretinide reduced risk: 35 percent less in women under age 50, and 50 percent less in women under age

40.[9] The drug's protective benefit continued even after women stopped taking it. Impressive results, yet the medication actually increased risk for a second breast cancer in women age 55 and older. The study didn't include previvors, so researchers can't conclude that fenretinide prevents breast cancer in these women.

Statins

Millions of people around the world take statins to reduce cholesterol and lower their risk of heart attack. One observational, retrospective study found that women who took statins regularly were 51 percent less likely to develop breast cancer.[10] Researchers can't be certain statins get the credit—in other studies involving women of average risk, these drugs haven't shown a protective effect. Studies are under way to determine whether statins reduce risk for high-risk women.

Deslorelin

Removing the ovaries lowers breast cancer risk, particularly in women with BRCA mutations. Deslorelin acetate prevents ovaries from producing estrogen, fueling speculation that it may also protect against breast cancer. Unlike surgical removal of the ovaries, deslorelin's effect is reversible: once a woman stops taking it, her ovaries begin making estrogen again. One preliminary study of deslorelin in premenopausal women with BRCA mutations showed it decreased breast density, which is linked to lower breast cancer risk and improved detection of early stage tumors by mammography. This research is encouraging; more study is needed to determine whether deslorelin lowers breast cancer risk.

Bisphosphonates

Data from the Women's Health Initiative show that women who took oral bisphosphonates, bone-building medications used to treat osteoporosis, were 30 to 40 percent less likely to develop invasive hormone receptor-positive breast cancer than women who didn't take the medication.[11] Surprisingly, women who used either Fosamax, Actonel, or Boniva were 58 percent more likely to develop DCIS. Researchers aren't sure why or how this occurs. They theorize that the medication somehow delays DCIS from evolving into invasive cancer. That would explain why there were fewer invasive cancers and more DCIS during the eight years of the study. An Israeli study found similar results, showing that women who took bisphosphonates for at least one year were 39 percent less likely to develop breast cancer than women who never took the drugs.[12] Whether these drugs can be used proactively remains to be seen and requires clinical trials. Bisphosphonates are associated with an increased risk of femur (thigh bone) fractures and esophageal cancer; the FDA now requires this information to be included in the safety labels of these medications.

Metformin

The most common medication used to treat type 2 diabetes may also inhibit breast cancer cell growth. Increasingly, evidence is mounting that metformin not only reduces blood sugar and insulin levels, it may improve breast cancer outcomes or even decrease risk for new breast tumors. In one study of 22,621 European women with type 2 diabetes, those who took metformin for five years or more had about 60 percent less chance of developing breast cancer compared to those who used other medications.[13] Metformin may act on both ER+ and triple-negative breast cancers, raising the possibility that it could be equally effective for BRCA1 and BRCA2 mutation carriers.

EXPERT VIEW: Could PARP Inhibitors Prevent Cancer?

BY JUDY E. GARBER, M.D., M.P.H.

A new class of targeted drugs called PARP inhibitors (PARPis) holds promise for treating BRCA-related cancers and may prove effective for preventing them as well. PARPis block poly (ADP-ribose) polymerase proteins, enzymes used by cells to repair certain kinds of damaged DNA. BRCA-related tumors, because they have lost a working copy of the gene, have a defect in one of the pathways cells use to fix those errors. In clinical trials involving patients with advanced BRCA-associated breast and ovarian cancer, PARPis given alone or combined with some chemotherapy drugs have reduced tumor size, although they have so far not cured women with advanced disease.

The medications appear to cause few side effects, even when patients are very ill. Researchers plan to study whether PARPis can safely reduce the chance of breast cancer in high-risk women. They hope to determine whether the medications can destroy damaged cells before they grow out of control and evolve into cancer, while leaving normal, healthy cells intact. To make sure the medications have a detectable effect on breast tissue and are safe, they will first be tested only briefly in BRCA mutation carriers who do not have cancer but who intend to have mastectomies, so their tissue can be studied after surgery. We need to ensure that PARP inhibitors are safe and effective before we can add them to the list of risk-reduction options.

Chemoprevention for Ovarian Cancer

Developing better methods for ovarian cancer risk management is challenging. We aren't yet able to find it in its early stages, and learning how to prevent it, short of removing the ovaries, requires more long-term research with large groups of women.

Oral Contraceptives

Fifty years after the Pill gave women control over their own fertility, it's now helping to protect them against ovarian cancer. Several studies show that oral contraceptives lower the risk for malignant ovarian tumors by up to 50 percent in women of average risk and in those with BRCA mutations.[14] Oral contraceptives are not without side effects, however, including a slightly increased risk for blood clots. Some research suggests that women with BRCA mutations who used oral contraceptives before 1975 (when estrogen content was much higher), before age 30, or for five or more years had greater risk for early onset breast cancer compared to BRCA mutation carriers who never used the medications. These studies aren't conclusive, and because much of the risk for ovarian cancer occurs after age 35, some experts recommend taking oral contraceptives to reduce risk only after age 30.

Analgesics

Research to determine whether analgesics decrease ovarian cancer risk is mixed. The Nurses' Health Study found a risk reduction associated with NSAIDs. These observational studies didn't specifically review ovarian cancer risk in women with BRCA mutations.

Fenretinide

The same medication that may reduce premenopausal breast cancer risk may also be an effective method of ovarian cancer chemoprevention in the high-risk population, at least while it's taken—a small study in breast cancer survivors who took fenretinide to prevent recurrence found it also reduced ovarian cancer risk during the five years women took it. The risk-lowering effect didn't continue once the medication was stopped.[15] The study also suggested that this protective effect may be stronger in women with BRCA mutations than in women with sporadic breast cancer. Current clinical trials are studying whether fenretinide can lower the odds of developing ovarian cancer in women with BRCA mutations.

INSURANCE AND PAYMENT ISSUES

Most insurance companies pay for FDA-approved medications to prevent cancer. If you participate in a clinical trial, there is usually no cost for any studied medications. Effective 2014, federal law will require new insurance plans to cover your expense for participating in a clinical trial for cancer or other life-threatening illness and provide normal health care during your participation. If you're uninsured or can't pay for chemoprevention medications, some pharmaceutical companies offer patient assistance programs if you meet certain criteria. Check the companies' websites for details.

THE FORCE PERSPECTIVE: WHY DON'T MORE WOMEN EMBRACE CHEMOPREVENTION?

Cancer experts expected a rush of high-risk women to get tamoxifen once it was approved by the FDA. That never happened. Despite the effectiveness of tamoxifen and raloxifene, many women don't consider the side effects to be worth the 50 percent risk reduction. In a FORCE poll of previvors who still have their natural breasts, fewer than 10 percent had ever taken tamoxifen. The same was true for raloxifene. About 66 percent indicated that their doctors had never recommended tamoxifen to reduce their risk. Forty percent were willing to participate in research to test new methods of chemoprevention. That's important, because more BRCA-specific research is needed. Perhaps doctors would recommend preventive drugs more frequently if they could more accurately predict how well the medicines would work for high-risk women, particularly those with BRCA mutations.

WHAT TO REMEMBER ABOUT CHEMOPREVENTION

- Chemoprevention drugs don't guarantee you won't develop cancer, but they improve your odds of staying cancer free.
- The degree of protection depends on your individual level of risk and other factors.
- Understand and weigh the potential benefits and risks of chemoprevention drugs before deciding which, if any, is right for you.
- Recommendations for chemoprevention will likely change as more research is performed.

Follow the status of chemoprevention clinical trials online at the National Institutes of Health website (clinicaltrials.gov) or at the Coalition of Cancer Cooperative Groups (www.cancertrialshelp.org).

Read more about the STAR trial (www.cancer.gov/clinicaltrials /noteworthy-trials/star), the Women's Health Initiative (www.whiscience .org), and the Nurses' Health Study (www.channing.harvard.edu/nhs).

Chapter 10 Mastectomy for

Risk Reduction and

Treatment

MASTECTOMY (surgically removing the breasts) is sometimes the wisest course of treatment. *Unilateral* mastectomy removes one breast; *bilateral* mastectomy removes both. Although aggressive and drastic, prophylactic bilateral mastectomy (PBM)—removing both healthy breasts—is the most effective way to reduce your chance of developing breast cancer.

Reducing Cancer Risk by Removing the Breasts

PBM lowers breast cancer risk by 90 percent or more.[1] Regardless of its risk-reducing efficiency, removing a healthy breast to avoid breast cancer is a tough decision, and it isn't acceptable to everyone. For some women, removing breasts to prevent cancer they may never develop seems extreme. For others, the decision remedies the concern they feel, especially if they've seen loved ones wage war against breast cancer. Individual circumstances and tolerance for risk greatly influence one's decision. Two women of the same age and same risk may approach the option of mastectomy differently. One might decide to delay or forego mastectomies, while the other may feel a more urgent need to address her risk surgically. Whatever your circumstances, mastectomy is irreversible. Have a clear sense of your own risk, speak with your healthcare team, and think carefully before deciding if it's the best risk management option for you.

Until the 1970s, a woman with breast cancer had one treatment option: the deforming and debilitating Halsted radical mastectomy that removed her entire breast, including skin and underlying pectoral muscle. Today, mastectomy is rarely that extreme, unless a woman has a tumor in the chest wall. When invasive cancer is found, a modified radical mastectomy removes the entire breast, including the nipple, areola, and some underarm lymph nodes. A total mastectomy removes breast tissue and spares the lymph nodes for high-risk women who choose preventive surgery.

WHAT ABOUT SENSATION?

Lost sensation is an unfortunate side effect of mastectomy that can't be restored, even after reconstruction, and even if most of the breast skin and nipples are spared. Most feeling is lost because the nerves are severed when tissue is removed. Generally, more sensation remains around the outer parts of the breast; the area around the areola and nipple usually remains numb. Some sensation may return after a year or more as nerves regenerate. Some women say they retain much of their sensation after mastectomy. Most feel pressure or nothing at all.

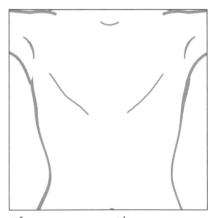

After mastectomy without reconstruction

If you're facing mastectomy, you have a lot to think about. But it's the best time to consider whether you want to have new breasts created, because certain mastectomy procedures accommodate shorter, less-visible incisions for immediate reconstruction when both surgeries are performed during a single visit to the operating room. If you have immediate reconstruction, you enter the operating room with your own breasts, which are removed and then rebuilt while you're under anesthesia, so you wake up with new breasts in place. If you decide not to have reconstruction, as many women do, your surgeon will make two incisions from side to side across the entire breast. He'll remove your breast tissue, nipple, areola, and most of the breast skin, and then suture the edges of the incisions together in a straight line. If you have delayed reconstruction in the future, your mastectomy scar will remain on your reconstructed breast. Doctors often don't inform mastectomy patients, particularly older women, of their reconstructive options. That's unfortunate, because all women deserve to be treated as individuals and make their own decisions about what's in their best interest. It pays to do your own research.

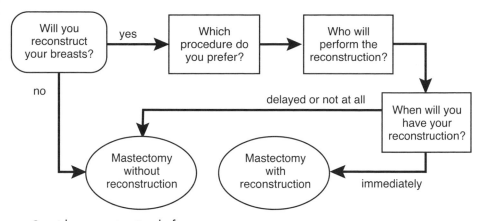

Consider reconstruction before your mastectomy

Sampling Lymph Nodes

The lymphatic system, including lymph nodes, vessels, and fluid, is a critical part of the immune system. Lymph fluid circulates through the body, collecting bacteria, viruses, dead blood cells, and other unwanted materials, including cancer cells. Lymph nodes filter out these pathogens, returning cleansed lymph to the circulatory system. You've probably noticed the glands in your neck (they're really lymph nodes) swell when you get strep throat. That's because white blood cells within the nodes are trying to clear away infection-causing cells.

Whenever invasive breast cancer is diagnosed, lymph nodes in the axilla (underarm) are sampled to see if they contain malignant cells. Any nodes that look or feel cancerous are removed during mastectomy in a procedure called *axillary lymph node dissection.* This is an important step in staging cancer and planning treatment, because if cancer cells are found in the lymph nodes, it indicates that more treatment may be needed. For most women diagnosed with early stage cancer, when lymph node involvement is unlikely, less invasive *sentinel node biopsy* is usually performed instead. By injecting a blue dye or radioactive tracer (or both) into the breast, the surgeon can follow the lymph system from the tumor to the sentinel node (usually the node nearest to the tumor). If the sentinel node contains cancer cells, an axillary dissection is then performed to determine whether other nodes are affected. If the sentinel node is free of cancer cells, the patient is spared the more invasive axillary dissection. Having negative nodes means cancer is less likely to have spread beyond the breast or to return after treatment.

Lymph nodes aren't usually removed during PBM, because previvors are assumed to be free of breast cancer. In a small percentage of high-risk women, cancer is discovered during prophylactic mastectomy, and some surgeons perform sentinel node biopsy as a precautionary measure. If invasive breast cancer is found during PBM, some underarm lymph nodes are sampled.

Skin-Sparing Procedures

If you have mastectomy with immediate reconstruction, your breast surgeon will perform a skin-sparing procedure to remove as much breast tissue as possible while leaving most of the skin in place to hold your new breast. Typically, the nipple and areola are cut away and the breast tissue is then removed through the opening. If you have a large tumor or large breasts, your surgeon may need to make an additional vertical or horizontal incision from the nipple. Skin-sparing mastectomies aren't recommended for women who have cancer in or very near the breast skin.

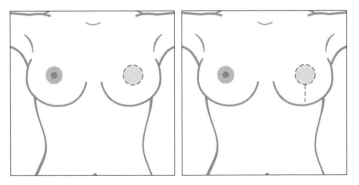

Skin-sparing incisions

Nipple-Sparing Mastectomy

Removing the nipple has traditionally been considered a mandatory part of the mastectomy procedure. Since breast cancer rarely occurs afterward, nipple-sparing mastectomies, particularly prophylactic mastectomies, are now more common. A nipple-sparing mastectomy conserves the areola, nipple, and most of the breast skin and is generally considered effective for preventive mastectomy. Some breast cancer patients may also be candidates, depending on the size and location of their tumor, although many physicians still consider nipple-sparing to be experimental. Individuals with tumors that are very large, aggressive, or close to (or within) the skin or nipples aren't candidates for this operation. Unlike traditional mastectomy, a nipple-sparing procedure eliminates the need to create and tattoo a new nipple, and the outcome is often more satisfying than a breast with recreated nipples and tattooed areolas.

Nipple-sparing incisions can be placed in several locations on the breast. Incisions made around the areola risk more tissue loss, while incisions below the breast or along the side leave better blood flow to the nipple. The nipple and areola remain attached to the breast skin and its blood supply during the operation to increase the chance of healing and retained sensation. The breast tissue beneath the nipple is removed, and a sample is then reviewed by a pathologist before the mastectomy is

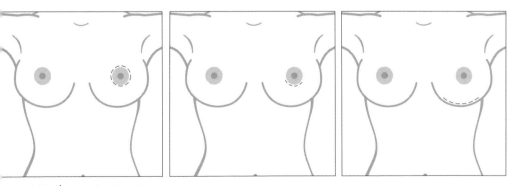

Nipple-sparing incisions

completed—it's called a frozen section because the pathologist freezes and stains the tissue with dye to examine it microscopically. If the sample contains cancerous cells, the nipple and areola are removed. Some surgeons prefer to remove the nipple and areola during surgery, and later graft them back onto the breast.

Women sometimes feel strongly about keeping their nipples, yet it often proves disappointing. Without the infrastructure of nerves and tissue, regrafted nipples may not respond to sensation or cold and often have little or no feeling. Sometimes the nipple-areola complex is poorly positioned on the new breast (particularly with large or drooping breasts) or suffers necrosis (tissue death from insufficient blood supply) and must be removed anyway. The remaining nipple may be flattened, although it can be plumped somewhat with soft tissue fillers.

EXPERT VIEW: Blood Flow Is Critical for Nipple-Sparing Mastectomy

BY DAVID J. WINCHESTER, M.D., F.A.C.S.

One of the concerns with nipple-sparing mastectomy is that much of the blood supply to the nipple is derived from the underlying breast tissue and not the surrounding skin. It is necessary to divide these blood vessels to separate the tissue from the overlying nipple. Everyone has different anatomic variations; until this step is taken, it's difficult to determine whether the nipple will survive. If it can immediately get enough blood flow from the surrounding skin, it will remain healthy. When the incision is placed right next to the nipple, a significant portion of the necessary blood flow is temporarily divided; blood flow is usually better when the incision is placed either along the outer breast or the lower portion of the breast. Most incisions are concealed from view, and the burden of cancer risk is dramatically reduced. Although there are other considerations in predicting a successful outcome with a nipple-sparing mastectomy, it's considered a safe option for women, and patient satisfaction is very high.

MY STORY: My Nipple-Sparing Decision

I'm happy with my decision to keep my nipples. They don't look perfect: the areolae are indented on the top, just inside where the incision was made, and that makes the projecting part of the nipple angle out and up. Perhaps this will change with time, as my surgery was only three weeks ago. They do have sensation, and that's important to me. I'm pretty sure I wouldn't have any sensation if I had lost my nipples. Of course, it's hard for me to compare this with how I would feel with reconstructed nipples, since I don't know that experience. Maybe I would be just as happy or happier. —SUZI

Subcutaneous Mastectomy

Subcutaneous (which is also called sub-mammary) mastectomy removes most breast tissue but leaves behind more than other types of mastectomy procedures. Subcutaneous incisions are often made in the breast fold, leaving the skin, areola, and nipple intact without any visible scarring. Because more tissue and nerves are left behind, you'll probably have more sensation around your nipple than someone who has traditional or nipple-sparing mastectomy. Women with large tumors, cancer in the breast skin, or tumors under or near the nipple or areola aren't candidates for subcutaneous mastectomy. Not all breast surgeons perform this procedure.

Areola-Sparing Mastectomy

Some surgeons offer mastectomy that removes the nipple and preserves the are-

HOW MUCH RISK REMAINS?

Mastectomy reduces lifetime breast cancer risk by 90 percent or more. If your estimated absolute lifetime risk is now 64 percent, it will be just 6.4 percent or less after PBM, lower than the risk of women who don't have a mutation. Mastectomy doesn't completely eliminate breast cancer risk, because it's not possible to remove every bit of breast tissue or every breast cell. The amount of tissue removed and the risk that remains may vary between procedures and among surgeons. No trials have compared one form of mastectomy to another. There isn't enough research, particularly among BRCA carriers, to know the remaining risk after prophylactic subcutaneous mastectomy—reported cases of subsequent breast cancer are low.

(continued)

No matter which mastectomy procedure you choose, enough tissue is removed so that mammography is no longer required. For high-risk women, some physicians recommend yearly breast MRI to scan remaining tissue, although no data supports this approach. It's important to perform monthly BSE to discover any lump or irregularity as soon as possible. Postmastectomy breast cancer may appear anywhere below the remaining skin or areola. (If breast cancer occurs after mastectomy, it usually reappears close to the original location of the tumor.) Firmly examine the area around your breasts, up to the collarbone and down below the ribs, looking for hard pea-sized bumps or anything that feels or looks unusual.

ola. Research specific to this procedure is lacking; the risk of developing breast cancer after an areola-sparing mastectomy may be similar to other nipple-sparing operations. Unlike nipples, areolas are just skin, without ductal tissue, where cancer is more likely to develop. If you want to have new nipples created, you'll need another small operation.

Treating Breast Cancer with Mastectomy

Treating breast cancer always involves some type of surgery. A partial mastectomy called lumpectomy is often sufficient to eliminate an early stage tumor and enough adjacent tissue so the surrounding margins are clear of cancerous cells. Breast-conserving lumpectomy preserves the remaining breast and is usually followed by radiation at the tumor site to destroy any remaining cancer cells. In most cases, lumpectomy with radiation is as effective against recurrence as mastectomy. However, mastectomy is often recommended when any of the following occur:

- Your cancer appears in two or more areas of the breast.
- Your surgeon is unable to get clear margins with lumpectomy.
- Removing a large lump will disfigure your small breast.
- You're pregnant.
- Your breast or chest was previously irradiated.
- You can't have radiation due to lupus or other connective tissue disease.
- You have a BRCA mutation, a strong family history of breast cancer, LCIS, or other indicator that you're at high risk.

For most patients with early stage tumors under 4 centimeters (about the size of a walnut), lumpectomy and radiation is as effective as mastectomy, with similar survival rates.[2] Yet candidates for lumpectomy frequently choose mastectomy instead. If both surgeries are equally effective, why wouldn't women keep their own breasts? Once a woman deals with the physical and emotional ups and downs of breast cancer, it's understandable why she might worry about a new diagnosis. The priority for most patients is to aggressively eliminate future risk in either breast, and they might choose mastectomy instead of lumpectomy for several reasons. Not all patients have radiation facilities nearby or can accommodate weeks of radiation appointments. Some say they would just as soon not face the ordeal of diagnosis and treatment again later in life, and mastectomy gives them a greater peace of mind and sense of safety.

High-risk women have another reason to choose mastectomy. In addition to risk in the opposite breast, a growing body of research shows that women with hereditary breast cancers are more likely to develop a new cancer in the same breast, even after lumpectomy and radiation.[3] A retrospective international study involving hundreds of women with BRCA-related breast cancer showed that survival was the same whether the women had lumpectomy and radiation or mastectomy, but the lumpectomy and radiation patients were four to five times more likely to develop a new cancer in the treated breast.[4] Adjuvant chemotherapy after lumpectomy and radiation lowered their risk for a new breast cancer in the treated breast.

Contralateral Mastectomy

Faced with the loss of one breast, more women, especially younger women, are choosing contralateral prophylactic mastectomy to remove their opposite healthy breast as well. Rates of contralateral mastectomy more than doubled in the United States between 1998 and 2003.[5] The NCCN doesn't routinely recommend contralateral mastectomy for women with sporadic tumors, because it hasn't been shown to improve survival. The risk for a new tumor in the opposite breast—less than 1 percent per year—isn't considered to be high. Research shows that women with BRCA1 mutations develop contralateral breast cancer almost five times more often and BRCA2 carriers about three times more often than women with sporadic breast cancer.[6] Still, it's more than some women can accept. Removing both breasts puts to rest concerns about facing a new diagnosis, and for some women, knowing both breasts can be reconstructed at the same time somewhat alleviates their concerns about mastectomy. Increasing use of MRIs before surgery to screen the opposite breast contributes to more contralateral surgeries. Women who have MRIs before a unilateral mastectomy are twice as likely to opt for contralateral mastectomy than those who don't (even though MRIs produce many false positives).[7] Sometimes women who need mastectomy to treat cancer in one breast decide to remove the opposite breast as well, because reconstructing both breasts at the same time results in better symmetry.

NCCN guidelines suggest contralateral mastectomy be considered on a case-by-case basis for high-risk women, particularly BRCA carriers.

Who Should Perform Your Surgery?

If you're shopping for a physician to perform your mastectomy, choose a general surgeon, breast surgeon, or surgical oncologist who performs mastectomies regularly. If you're considering nipple-sparing mastectomies, ask how many the surgeon has performed. What's his rate of success or failure in keeping the nipple? Ask to speak with other prophylactic mastectomy patients and see photos of their results. In some parts of the country, it may be difficult to find surgeons who offer nipple-sparing mastectomy. If you're pursuing prophylactic surgery, you have more time to research and interview several surgeons before deciding who is best for you.

Risks and Recovery

Most women recover from mastectomy without serious problems. Like all operations, however, problems can occur and sometimes require additional medical intervention (see table 9).

Table 9. Risks of mastectomy surgery

More common issues	Less common issues
Infection	Blood loss
Fluid or blood buildup at the surgical site (seroma/hematoma)	Blood clots
	Long-term postoperative pain
Delayed healing	Hard scar tissue at mastectomy site
	Shoulder pain or stiffness
	Nipple loss

Infection

Developing an infection after mastectomy or any surgery is uncommon, but it happens. Report immediately any unusual redness, swelling, or feeling of heat in the breast (beyond that caused by normal healing) to your doctor. In most cases, a round of antibiotics will clear up the problem. Broader infections can be more difficult and may delay healing.

Seroma or Hematoma

If fluid or blood collects deep in the incision site, it's usually absorbed by the body over time. Larger seromas or hematomas can cause swelling, bruising, or pain that requires medical attention. If draining the area with a needle doesn't resolve the problem, surgery may be needed.

Postmastectomy Pain Syndrome

There's often surprisingly little pain after a mastectomy, especially when no reconstruction is involved. Routine postoperative pain as tissue and nerves heal is handled with prescription or over-the-counter medication. Mild to serious pain may occur after you've healed, especially if you're young or have lymph nodes removed. Some women report sharp, burning, or shooting pain in the underarm, chest wall, or shoulder, or

DEALING WITH DRAINS

Ask women what they found most uncomfortable about post-op recovery and they'll probably say surgical drains. These small plastic bulbs connect to a long thin tube that is sutured under the skin to collect fluid and blood at the incision site. Drains are annoying, though without them, excess fluid can build up, delay healing, and invite infection. They're awkward under clothes and in the shower, and can be painful if you pull the tube where it enters the skin. Drains remain in place for a few days to weeks after surgery (longer when axillary dissection or reconstruction is performed) and are removed once postsurgery fluid buildup has sufficiently decreased. Removing drains is usually painless, and most women are happy to have them gone.

develop *postmastectomy pain syndrome* (PMPS), chronic pain that is usually a by-product of nerves severed during mastectomy and that can persist indefinitely. PMPS can be difficult to diagnose, because physicians may initially assume it's normal postsurgical pain associated with healing. It can also be difficult to treat. Yoga, acupuncture, and massage by a knowledgeable physical therapist can provide relief. If your pain persists, you may need to consult with a pain specialist.

Lymphedema

Studies suggest that up to 20 percent of patients who have breast cancer surgery that includes axillary dissection at some point experience lymphedema, a mild to serious long-term complication caused by fluid buildup and swelling in the arm, hand, or chest wall and is more common when axillary nodes are removed. Lymphedema can appear any time after surgery, but once diagnosed, it's often treatable. Taking lifelong precautionary measures can lessen the risk for developing symptoms. If nodes were removed from one underarm, always use the opposite arm for injections, blood pressure readings, and drawing blood. Wearing a lymphatic sleeve prescribed by your doctor will usually help to prevent or decrease swelling. Therapeutic massage by a qualified physical therapist can minimize swelling and relieve pressure in the arm. Gentle strength training directed by a physical therapist who has special training about lymphedema can reduce symptoms and their frequency.

INSURANCE AND PAYMENT ISSUES

Most insurance carriers now cover the cost of PBM with documentation provided by your doctor verifying your high-risk status. Before scheduling your mastectomy, be sure your surgeon and treatment facility are acceptable to your carrier. You're responsible for whatever normal copayments and deductibles apply according to the conditions of your policy: if you typically pay 20 percent of medical costs, you'll be required to do the same for your mastectomy. Federal law requires health policies that cover mastectomy to also pay for treatment for any related health problems, including lymphedema.

If you're uninsured, contact your local American Cancer Society or Susan G. Komen for the Cure affiliate about donated surgical services. Unfortunately, some companies still consider prophylactic mastectomy to be medically unnecessary and routinely deny such requests, even for women with high hereditary risk. If your insurance carrier refuses to cover your procedure, ask your doctor to write a supportive appeal letter explaining why mastectomy is necessary to reduce your extraordinary breast cancer risk.

THE FORCE PERSPECTIVE:

MASTECTOMY LOWERS RISK—DOES IT IMPROVE SURVIVAL?

Some women report that their healthcare professionals question the choice of PBM to reduce breast cancer risk because it hasn't been shown to improve survival. That seems to be contradictory, yet it's true. You might wonder how something that almost eliminates the possibility of cancer doesn't automatically ensure you'll live a longer life; however, research conducted in the last decade doesn't reflect improved survival after PBM. Mastectomy greatly improves your odds of never developing breast cancer or having to endure chemotherapy, radiation, or other treatment; it doesn't necessarily mean you'll live longer. Most high-risk women who are diagnosed early survive their breast cancer, and perhaps PBM simply doesn't improve an already strong survival rate. It's more likely that research following high-risk women after PBM hasn't studied them long enough. As more long-term studies follow women beyond ten years postsurgery, a survival benefit from PBM may emerge.

WHAT TO REMEMBER ABOUT MASTECTOMY

- Prophylactic bilateral mastectomy reduces up to 90 percent (or more) of breast cancer risk.
- Because it's not possible to totally remove all breast tissue, a small risk remains.
- Mastectomy eliminates much of the sensation in the breast.
- Ask your surgeon to describe the length and exact location of your incisions before your operation.

LEARN MORE ABOUT MASTECTOMY

Visit the FORCE message boards and mastectomy photo gallery (www.facingourrisk.org) to learn from other women who have had mastectomy. Check the "Pearls of Wisdom" section for before and after surgery tips.

Dr. Susan Love's Breast Book, by Susan Love, M.D., is a comprehensive guide to understanding breast conditions and how they're treated.

The Breast Reconstruction Guidebook, by Kathy Steligo, includes several informative chapters about mastectomy.

The National Lymphedema Network (www.lymphnet.org) provides education and support for lymphedema patients.

Chapter 11   Reconstruction

New Breasts after
Mastectomy

RECONSTRUCTION AFTER MASTECTOMY replaces the volume and shape
of your breasts. In the hands of a gifted plastic surgeon, reconstruction
isn't just an operation, it's art. Surgical techniques have greatly improved
in the last decade, particularly benefiting women who have PBM with
immediate reconstruction. The goal is no longer to simply restore your
profile in clothes, but to make you look as natural as possible with or
without clothes.

Traditional reconstruction procedures involve two or more operations over several months. The initial surgery forms breast mounds
without nipples, replacing tissue removed during mastectomy with
implants or *flaps* (sections of tissue from your back, abdomen, thigh,
or buttocks). This first stage is the most complex and involves the most
recovery. Depending on the procedure, a shorter revision surgery then
refines the shape and size of your new breasts and adds nipples. Finally,
optional tattooing adds color to the nipple and areola.

Some women prefer not to have reconstruction. Those who do have
several options, each with advantages and disadvantages. If you're considering reconstruction, it's important to learn about your choices;
decide which, if any, is best for you; and select a surgeon who is experienced and skilled in that procedure (see table 10, page 131).

Delaying Reconstruction to Complete Breast Cancer Treatment

Although most women can have immediate reconstruction, your
oncologist may recommend a delay of six months to a year to avoid the

possibility of infection or healing issues before you complete chemotherapy or radiation. A temporary implant called an expander can be placed during your mastectomy and slowly inflated during your chemo treatments. In six to twelve weeks after your last treatment, when your immune system is fully recovered, your expanders can then be replaced with implants and your new nipples created. Or you can wait and have delayed reconstruction once you've completed treatment. Tissue flaps are major surgery; if that is your preferred method of reconstruction, you may have to wait until you've completed chemotherapy.

Reconstruction after radiation is more difficult, because the skin and blood supply are damaged by the treatment. Implant reconstruction after radiation has a particularly high potential for complications or loss of the implant. Sometimes the remaining breast skin is too thin and fragile for the implant process, and *extrusion* (the implant breaks through the skin) can occur. It sometimes works, especially if the skin is expanded very slowly. If it's damaged extensively and doesn't expand or the implant fails, a tissue flap is the only remaining reconstructive option. If you have your heart set on implant reconstruction, some surgeons will place an expander during mastectomy, quickly complete expansion, and exchange it for an implant before radiation.

Alternatively, saline can be removed from an expander before radiation, then refilled after the last treatment. If you need radiation after mastectomy, tissue flap reconstruction usually produces better results. Flap reconstruction may also be difficult after radiation, because the blood supply to the new breast is compromised. The risk of necrosis is higher, but in most cases, it isn't a serious problem.

SYMMETRY AFTER UNILATERAL RECONSTRUCTION

If you have unilateral mastectomy and reconstruction, matching your reconstructed breast to your natural breast can be challenging. It's somewhat easier to create the new breast with a tissue flap and, if necessary, then augment, reduce, or lift the opposite breast to match. Each of these procedures involves surgery, incisions, and scarring on the healthy breast. Be sure you understand what each modification entails before scheduling your surgery.

Living with a Flat Chest

If you choose not to reconstruct your breasts, as many women do, your chest will be flat after mastectomy. You might be just fine with this, especially if you've always had very small breasts or don't want to have additional surgery. If you decide against reconstruction but want to fill out your clothes, you can use *prostheses*, breast forms made of cotton, foam, latex, or silicone that stick to your chest or fit into a pocket in your bra. Wearing a prosthesis can also help to provide balance when trying to fit into clothes after unilateral mastectomy, or between mastectomy and delayed reconstruction.

Prostheses come in a variety of shapes, weights, and prices. Silicone is the most expensive because it has a consistency that is most like a natural breast. It's important to have a qualified fitter in a mastectomy boutique or department store help to fit you correctly. Visit tlcdirect. org, a website maintained by the American Cancer Society, for more information about breast prostheses.

MY STORY: My Breasts Don't Define Me

I chose no reconstruction for a simple reason: I wanted to be done with surgery. Part of me will always miss my breasts, but they don't define me, and reconstruction would not have given them back. One breast was removed due to invasive ductal breast cancer, and I chose the fastest surgery—reconstruction would have meant waiting for the plastic surgeon's schedule and a longer recovery. The other breast was removed a year later, along with my ovaries, after I learned I was BRCA1 positive and diagnosed with leukemia. I then opted for no recon because I didn't want to risk infection, reconstruction failure, or additional surgeries. For me, coming to terms with my new reality meant accepting that my own breasts were gone. I knew if I ever changed my mind, reconstruction would still be an option. Six years later, I haven't changed my mind. I am undeniably different, but I'm still me. I have no regrets about foregoing reconstruction. My choice may not have been right for everyone. It was simply the right one for me.   —LISA

Saline and Silicone Implants

Refilling the breast skin with saline or silicone implants is the quickest route to reconstruction, involving the shortest surgery and recovery. Implants come in different sizes and widths and are either round or anatomically shaped. Which is used is mostly determined by your anatomy. Saline implants are silicone shells filled with salt water. They're firmer than silicone gel implants, which are softer and feel more like natural breast tissue. Ask to hold and feel both before deciding which you prefer. You're a candidate for implant reconstruction if you're not excessively obese, don't have advanced disease, and haven't had multiple infections or surgeries at your mastectomy site.

Most implant reconstruction involves two phases. Expanders are first placed into pockets created under the pectoralis muscles and are gradually inflated with saline over several weeks in your surgeon's office. Your muscles and skin stretch each time more saline is added. Each of these "fill" appointments takes just minutes. Afterward, you'll feel tightness until your muscles and skin stretch again to accommodate the newly added saline. Some women find this process very uncomfortable; others sail through it without a second thought. Over-the-counter pain medications or prescribed muscle relaxants, if needed, make the expander process easier. In a few weeks, the pocket and breast skin are sufficiently stretched to accommodate your implants. The fully inflated expanders then typically stay in place for

IS SILICONE SAFE?

Despite past controversies, implants are generally considered to be safe, and newer silicone gel is believed to be less likely to rupture or bleed to surrounding tissue. (Preliminary research suggests that women with breast implants may have a very low but increased risk for anaplastic large cell lymphoma, a rare type of non-Hodgkin's lymphoma.) As a condition of approval, the FDA recommends biennial breast MRI beginning three years after reconstruction with silicone implants. (Insurance doesn't usually cover this cost.) By law, before surgery, your plastic surgeon should provide a copy of the package insert that describes implant safety and study data. Ask for it if you don't receive it, or read the data on the manufacturer's website.

Source: Federal Drug Administration, "Anaplastic Large Cell Lymphoma," www .fda.gov/MedicalDevices/Productsand MedicalProcedures/ImplantsandProsthe tics/BreastImplants/ucm239995.htm.

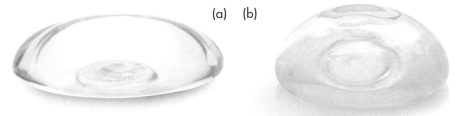

(a) (b)

Round moderate-profile (a) and high-profile (b) implants. Images provided by Mentor Worldwide LLC.

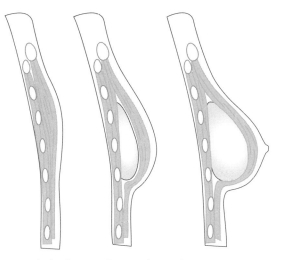

Expanders slowly stretch the breast skin and muscle

at least three months before being replaced with implants that fit your anatomy and your desired size—this is a shorter surgery, usually about an hour for each breast. Some surgeons use permanent expanders that are sealed in place and become the implant once the final breast size is achieved. The fill process is still required; an additional surgery to exchange the expander isn't needed. An excellent resource for anyone who wonders what the expansion process is like is Myself: Together Again (www.myselftogetheragain.org).

Direct-to-Implant Reconstruction

Single-stage implant reconstruction, also called *nonexpansive, direct-to-implant,* or *one-step* reconstruction, is the fastest way to recreate your

breasts with the least downtime. Combined with nipple-sparing mastectomy, direct-to-implant reconstruction places full-sized implants
immediately, avoiding expansion and additional operations. You leave
the operating room much as you entered: with fully formed breasts in
place. Unless a cosmetic or medical problem arises, you need no further
reconstructive procedures.

Direct-to-implant reconstruction uses patches of *acellular dermal
matrix* (donated human tissue that has been stripped of all its cells but
retains all the elements necessary to support new tissue growth) sewn
onto the muscle to form an immediate sling that holds the implant. It
also helps to camouflage implant edges that may be felt or seen under
the skin. Less frequently, surgeons place implants over the muscle if the
skin is thick enough. Sometimes one-step procedures turn into two-
step reconstruction if revisions are needed to fix a problem or asymmetry. Direct-to-implant surgeries are becoming more common, especially for women who have PBM, but most reconstructive surgeons still
prefer the traditional expansion method. If you're interested, be aware
that some surgeons now use acellular dermal matrix with traditional
expansion to better cover the expander and define the inframammary
fold under the breast. When a surgeon says he uses dermal matrix, ask
specifically if he uses it in a single-stage or expander process.

MY STORY: Better Than Ever

*My mother was diagnosed at age 59 with metastasized inflammatory
breast cancer, despite annual mammograms and ultrasound. She died the
next year. When my OB-GYN suggested I get tested for a BRCA mutation,
I refused. What would I do if I inherited this risk, worry even more about
getting breast cancer? The years passed, and finally, I felt I had to be tested,
only when I knew what to do if I was positive. Thankfully, I found the
FORCE message boards, where I read about women who had prophylactic
mastectomy and kept their nipples intact and had implants placed in a single surgery. For the first time, I felt hope. If I tested positive, I had an option
I could live with. Within three months of testing positive for a BRCA2*

mutation, I had nipple-sparing mastectomies with direct-to-implant reconstruction. It wasn't easy. Once I recovered, my body looked better than ever. This procedure gave me impetus to save my life, and I've never looked back. —ANDREA

Implants Aren't Permanent

No implant lasts forever. Eventually they all must be replaced for one reason or another: infection, a shift in position, or the wrong size or shape. Implants that leak or rupture must also be replaced. A saline implant rupture is obvious because the breast deflates (saline is harmlessly absorbed into the body). Silicone ruptures aren't as noticeable, because the implant retains its shape—hence the FDA recommendation for biennial MRI screenings. *Capsular contracture*—scar tissue that hardens and squeezes the implant, distorting breast shape and causing discomfort or pain—usually requires surgery to remove the scar tissue and replace the implant, and even with this surgery, the same thing may happen again. Some women need their implants replaced within a year of reconstruction; others have theirs for fifteen years or longer. According to American Society of Plastic Surgeons member reports, in 2009 more than sixteen thousand women had their breast implants removed after reconstruction.[1]

Implants are a good option for women who:

- haven't had radiation to the chest.
- don't mind having additional surgery to eventually replace the implants.
- don't want to endure a longer recovery from tissue flap surgery or don't want to scar another area of their body.

Options for Using Your Own Tissue

Tissue flaps (*autologous* breast reconstructions) are more technically challenging, requiring special surgical skills and involving a more intense recovery than implant reconstruction. Breasts made with your own living tissue feel soft and move more like your natural breasts. Like your own breasts, they fluctuate as you lose or gain weight. The total reconstruction timeline is often shorter: about three to five months instead of the six months or more required for the expansion method. Unlike traditional implants, flaps form full-size breasts during the initial operation. Later revision surgery refines the shape and creates the nipples. Unlike implant procedures, flap surgeries create scars and permanent numbness along the flap incision at both the breast and donor site. Women who are overly obese, smoke, are too thin, or have had previous surgery that interrupted the blood supply at the donor site may not be candidates for flap surgery.

Flaps are a good option for women who:

- want new breasts made of their own tissue.
- have previously had radiation to the chest or breast.
- don't want to risk problems inherent with implants or endure the expansion process.
- want to match one reconstructed breast to their other natural breast.

One disadvantage of flaps is the risk for necrosis, where some or all of the transplanted tissue dies from an inadequate blood supply. When a small area of necrosis occurs as a hard lump or an area that feels thickened, it may resolve on its own or require surgical removal. Rarely, an entire flap fails and must be replaced. When this does occur, it's usually within the first few days after reconstruction; necrosis sometimes occurs weeks or months after surgery. Fat necrosis usually isn't cause for concern, but any lumps or changes should be checked by your surgeon.

Three types of tissue flaps are used in breast reconstruction, depending on the type of blood flow provided to the new breast. *Attached flaps* use skin, fat, and muscle from the back (*latissimus dorsi* flap, often combined with an implant for more volume) or the abdomen (*transverse rectus abdominis myocutaneous*—TRAM flap). During a TRAM procedure, a flap of abdominal tissue and muscle is tunneled under the skin from the donor site to the chest and is shaped into a breast. Once in place, it remains connected to its original blood supply. You get a bonus with an abdominal flap: the procedure is the same as a tummy tuck, except the excess tissue is used to build your new breast. However, removing entire muscles can leave permanent weakness at the donor site. Abdominal weakness and hernia can be a problem after attached TRAM surgery, even though most surgeons reinforce the area with surgical mesh. You shouldn't have problems with routine movements, but you'll probably not be able to do sit-ups again. A latissimus dorsi flap doesn't usually affect movement or strength, because other muscles in the back compensate.

Free flaps are complete transplants of skin, fat, and a small portion of muscle surrounding the blood vessels. This is technically more demanding than implant or attached flap reconstruction, because the surgeon must transfer the flap from the donor site to the chest and use a surgical microscope to reconnect the blood vessels at the mastectomy site. Free flaps can be taken from the abdomen (free TRAM) or the buttock (free gluteal flap). Less frequently, flaps from the hip (*lateral transverse thigh flap*) or inner thigh (*transverse upper gracilis* or TUG) can be used. Unlike attached flap procedures, free flap surgeries remove only a portion of the muscle to build the breast, so recovery is usually shorter and less painful.

Perforator flaps represent the most sophisticated reconstruction process. These are longer surgeries, but because they use no muscle at all, they are less invasive and less painful. Perforator flaps require the most expertise and precision, and fewer surgeons have the necessary training, although more are learning. Once the plastic surgeon removes the flap of tissue, he must carefully extract blood vessels from the surrounding muscle and then reconnect them in the chest. The *deep inferior epigastric perforator* (DIEP) flap uses abdominal fatty tissue, leaving full abdominal strength, so recovery is quicker. The *superficial inferior epigastric artery* (SIEA) *perforator* is similar but uses the abdominal artery above the muscle, so there's no need to cut into the muscle. In most women, this artery is too small to provide adequate blood flow. Nor can it be used in women who have had hysterectomy or cesarean section.

When women don't have enough abdominal fat for reconstruction, the buttock is often an adequate resource. The *superior gluteal artery perforator* (SGAP) uses tissue from the top of the buttocks; the *inferior gluteal artery perforator* (IGAP) takes tissue from the lower buttocks. These are lengthy operations, because the patient has to be turned twice: first to harvest the buttock tissue after mastectomy, then again to transfer the flap to the chest. Most plastic surgeons don't perform GAP reconstruction; those who do usually perform only one side at a time, requiring patients to have two separate ten- to twelve-hour surgeries. A few surgeons, most of whom devote their practice exclusively to reconstruction, perform bilateral simultaneous GAP in eight or nine hours.

EXPERT VIEW: Effects of Fitness and Smoking on Surgery

BY MINAS CHRYSOPOULO, M.D.

Wounds need a lot of energy to heal well. Since energy only comes from food, it is vital for patients to eat a healthy diet before and after surgery: protein, zinc, and vitamins A and C are crucial for wound healing. The importance of healthy nutrition is emphasized by the link between obesity and postsurgery complications. Obese patients have much higher rates of infection, wound-healing problems, and hematomas and seromas compared to nonobese patients. Obese patients also have thicker fat layers with poorer blood supply. Blood flow and the amount of vital nutrients and oxygen reaching healing tissues is therefore less robust.

Staying well-hydrated before and after surgery—drinking eight (8-oz) glasses of water a day and avoiding caffeinated beverages—is also very important, as dehydration causes the skin and soft tissues to become dry, which inhibits healing. Smoking also negatively impacts healing. Nicotine shrinks blood vessels, depriving tissues of the nutrients and oxygen required for healing. At best, this slows the wound-healing process; at worst, smoking can cause wounds to break down. (Many smoking-cessation products also increase the risk of healing problems because they also contain nicotine!) Cigarette smoke contains carbon monoxide, which combines with blood cells, lowering the level of oxygen in the blood. Since oxygen is vital for healing, it is crucial to quit smoking before and after surgery to decrease the risk of healing complications. Finally, regular aerobic exercise improves healing after surgery and boosts the immune system. Regular exercise before and after surgery (once cleared by your surgeon) is encouraged.

Table 10. Comparing reconstructive techniques

	Expanders/implants	*Tissue flaps*
Surgery	Two short operations, 3–6 months apart*	Longer initial operation; shorter subsequent procedures
Anesthesia	General	General
Hospital stay	2–3 days when done with mastectomy; overnight if performed as separate surgery	4–7 days whether performed with mastectomy or as separate surgery
Nipple	Separate procedure*	Separate procedure*
Scars	At mastectomy site	At mastectomy and donor sites

Source: Reprinted with permission of the author from Kathy Steligo, *The Breast Reconstruction Guidebook* (San Carlos, Calif.: Carlo Press, 2003).
*Nipple-sparing mastectomies with immediate reconstruction generally involve one surgery.

Optional Last Steps: Adding Nipples and Areolas

If you don't have nipple-sparing mastectomy, once a reconstructed breast settles into its final position—at least three months after implant exchange surgery or during flap revision surgery—nipples can be added to your breast mound. Reconstructed nipples are optional; because they remain erect and don't react to cold or touch the way natural nipples do, some women forego this part of reconstruction. Reconstructed nipples look like the real thing, even if they don't respond in the same way. Most

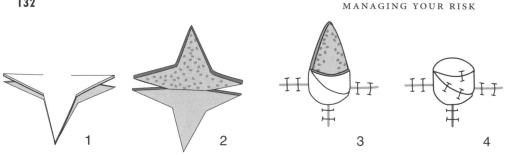

Creating a nipple from breast skin

surgeons free a small flap of breast skin, twist or fold it over to fashion it into a nipple, and suture it in place. Some surgeons prefer to graft skin from the inner thigh, labia, or back of the ear onto the breast. Newly created nipples can be up to 50 percent larger than the desired size because they shrink significantly as they heal.

The last reconstructive step is tattooing color to the new nipple and areola. This usually brings a sense of closure to the breast cancer and reconstruction experience. Once the nipple is created, your surgeon or medical aesthetician tints the areola and nipple or refers you to a professional tattoo artist who is experienced with reconstructive tattooing. (Women who prefer not to have reconstructed nipples sometimes simulate them with clever tattooing.) Because a reconstructed breast has little or no sensation, most women feel the tattooing more as pressure than pain. Tattoos lose much of their color after two or three years; tattooing them again restores their pigment.

Great Expectations: Surgery and Recovery

Most women are satisfied with their new breasts. Many aren't. It helps to start with realistic expectations and make sure you and your surgeon are on the same page about your results. Discuss every aspect of your reconstruction, explaining what type of implants you prefer, what size you want your new breasts to be (that should be your decision, not his), and how large your nipples should be. Ask what to expect from surgery

Table 11. Risks of reconstructive surgery

More common issues	*Less common issues*
Infection	Blood loss
Fluid or blood buildup at the surgical site (seroma/hematoma)	Blood clots
	Necrosis
Delayed healing	Loss of implant or flap
Postoperative pain	Long-term postoperative pain
Aesthetic issues	

and recovery and how he will handle any cosmetic or healing problems (see table 11). Leaving all the decisions up to your surgeon increases the chance you'll be surprised or unhappy with your breasts.

Most breast reconstructions require revision surgery, a secondary operation to fine tune or address asymmetry, poor positioning, or other cosmetic issues. It's a good idea to discuss these issues with your surgeon before your reconstruction, including the following aesthetic problems.

Cosmetic Issues

Let's face it. Most of us were not born with perfect breasts. Reconstruction probably won't give them to you either, yet it's an opportunity to reduce, enlarge, or otherwise cosmetically improve your breasts. If you have asymmetrical, almost-not-there, or large sagging breasts before mastectomy, your new breasts can resolve those issues. Swapping implants can improve rippling, wrinkles, or other visible cosmetic defects. Indentations or misshapen flaps can be enhanced with fat that is liposuctioned from somewhere else on your body.

Projection

Unless you have nipple-sparing mastectomy, you'll probably have less projection after reconstruction than before. Removing the nipple during mastectomy somewhat flattens the contour of the breast, like cutting a hole in a balloon and then restitching it. Talk to your surgeon about options for achieving the best possible projection.

Symmetry

Generally, natural breasts aren't exactly alike. They're often different sizes in different positions and may have misaligned nipples. When both breasts are reconstructed, it's easier to make them symmetrical because the surgeon is starting from a clean slate. When only one breast is reconstructed, you may need to augment, lift, or reduce your remaining healthy breast if you want to be symmetrical. This is especially true if your breast is reconstructed with an implant, which is likely to result in a high, perky breast that probably won't match your natural breast.

MY STORY: If I Had To Do It Over, I Would Do It Differently

Overall, I'm happy with my bilateral attached TRAM reconstruction. My breasts look and feel natural. If I were to do it over, I'd consider a different type of flap reconstruction. My surgeon told me that I wouldn't be able to do sit-ups anymore. I don't miss doing them, but I do sometimes miss my abdominal muscles. If I'm lying flat on my back, I feel like a beached whale, unable to move around easily. Most evenings I read in bed as I lean back on a wedge pillow. Each time I move around to adjust my position, I need to push against the bed with my hands because my remaining stomach muscles just can't do it. Something that was once effortless is now clumsy. Another effect of the muscle loss is that fat in my midriff pooches out instead of being held in by my muscles. This doesn't affect the way I function, but it affects my appearance and how I feel about myself.   —AMI

Choosing the Right Surgeon

Choosing the right plastic surgeon can make the difference between being satisfied and being disappointed. Someone who routinely does breast reconstruction is more likely to give you breasts you'll be happy with than someone who does implants or flaps a couple of times a month. Some surgeons devote their entire practice to reconstruction. Not all surgeons perform all procedures; they often recommend only the techniques they perform, so it's always a good idea to get a second and even a third opinion. The lone plastic surgeon in your area may only offer traditional expansion when you were hoping to take advantage of DIEP to get a nice tummy tuck and spare your abdominal muscles. You may have to travel (insurance doesn't cover the cost of travel or a hotel) to get the procedure you want.

SEVEN QUESTIONS FOR YOUR PLASTIC SURGEON

1. How many of these procedures have you done?
2. What should I expect from the surgery and recovery?
3. Realistically, what can I expect?
4. What risks or problems may occur?
5. What will you do to address them?
6. May I see your before-and-after photos?
7. May I speak to at least two of your patients who have had this same procedure?

INSURANCE ISSUES AND PAYMENT

Add up the cost for surgeons, anesthesiologists, and hospitals and you'll come up with a total that's beyond most people's financial means. The Women's Health and Cancer Rights Act (WHCRA) requires individual and group health plans, insurance companies, and health maintenance organizations (HMOs) that pay for mastectomy (most do) to also pay for breast prostheses, breast reconstruction, surgery to the other breast to achieve a symmetrical appearance, and treatment for complications from mastectomy or reconstruction. The law doesn't define how much or to whom insurers must pay, and many surgeons don't perform complex flap surgeries because insurance reimbursement is minimal. Despite the law, some insurance companies still routinely deny requests for reconstruction. If you belong to a managed care plan and choose an in-network facility and surgeon, you probably won't encounter problems gaining approval, and you'll limit your cost to standard copayments and deductibles, espe-cially if you choose implants with expansion, attached TRAM, or back flaps, which are more common. You'll more likely need to travel out-of-network for DIEP, GAP, or direct-to-implant reconstruction, because they're less common. You may need to convince your insurance company of why you need to go out-of-network. If you're lucky, the carrier will approve and refer you to an out-of-network surgeon, although you'll pay more, including airfare and hotel costs. You may also be responsible for balance billing (the difference between what the surgeon charges and what your insurance company pays); that's illegal in some states, so check with state officials to determine what applies.

Finalize all financing before your surgery date. Ask the billing special-ist in your plastic surgeon's office to help with insurance authorizations and claims. When denied, women often appeal, fight, escalate, and ulti-mately win, but it's a time-consuming and energy-draining experience. If you're without the means to pay for your reconstruction, canvas your local cancer center or several plastic surgeons to see if you're eligible for donated services.

THE FORCE PERSPECTIVE: CONSIDERING RECONSTRUCTION

Few decisions associated with HBOC are as multifaceted as those involv-ing reconstruction. Reconstructive choices and outcomes are the most com-mon topics on our message boards. We encourage our members to inter-view several surgeons, get as much input as possible, and see several finished reconstructions if they can. That's why women tell us the Show-and-Tell room at our annual conference is invaluable: there's nothing like seeing real results and talking to women who have already been through the process.

Consider the following before making your decision:

- What's your first choice for reconstruction?
- What types of reconstruction are available in your area?
- What types of reconstruction does the plastic surgeon who works with your breast surgeon perform?

- Are you willing to travel for surgery if your first choice isn't available locally?

At times during surgery or recovery, it may seem that you'll never be finished and that you might never again have a life of normal routine. Once your reconstruction is completed, you enter what FORCE members call "the All-Done Club." Hopefully, doctor appointments, pain, and recovery will then be behind you.

WHAT TO REMEMBER ABOUT RECONSTRUCTION

- Your breasts can be recreated with implants or your own tissue.
- Not all women are candidates for all procedures.
- Weigh the benefits and limitations of each procedure before selecting one.
- A plastic surgeon's skill and experience is the single most important factor in your overall satisfaction with your reconstruction.

LEARN MORE ABOUT RECONSTRUCTION

The Department of Labor, Pensions, and Welfare Benefits Administration (www.askebsa.dol.gov, or 800-998-7542) provides information about WHCRA and your rights to reconstruction.

Contact your Department of Health or Insurance Commissioner for information about your state's laws regarding reconstruction.

Visit the FORCE website to see postmastectomy and reconstruction photos (www.facingourrisk.org/reconstruction).

The Breast Reconstruction Guidebook, by Kathy Steligo, describes reconstructive techniques and issues in detail. The accompanying website (www.breastrecon.com) lists U.S. and Canadian surgeons who perform perforator flap and one-step implant procedures.

My Hope Chest (www.myhopechest.org) provides funding and resources for uninsured women to have breast reconstruction.

Chapter 12 Oophorectomy and

Other Risk-Reducing

Gynecologic Surgeries

IF YOU DEVELOP OVARIAN CANCER, your treatment will involve *oophorectomy*, surgery to remove your ovaries. If you have a BRCA mutation, the most effective way to lower your high risk for ovarian cancer is prophylactic bilateral salpingo-oophorectomy (BSO), removal of both ovaries and both fallopian tubes. (It's important to remove the fallopian tubes as well, because hereditary cancer may develop there.) Several studies of BRCA women, including the Prevention and Observation of Surgical Endpoints (PROSE) research funded by the National Institutes of Health, validate the significant risk-reducing effectiveness of BSO.[1] Experts recommend the surgery for women with BRCA mutations, ideally between the ages of 35 and 40 and when they have completed childbearing.

In women with BRCA mutations, BSO reduces the odds of dying from both breast and ovarian cancer, and decreases overall risk for dying prematurely. BSO also cuts your breast cancer risk in half.[2] If you develop breast cancer, it reduces your odds for a second diagnosis by half as well.[3] (See table 12.)

It may seem logical that removing the ovaries and tubes would reduce all risk for ovarian and fallopian tube cancer, but the facts are a

Table 12. Risk reduction from BSO before natural menopause

	Estimated risk reduction (%)
Ovarian / fallopian tube / primary peritoneal cancer	80 or more
Breast cancer	50
Contralateral breast cancer	50

bit more complicated. After BSO, 2 to 6 percent lifetime risk remains—much less than your lifetime risk if you keep your ovaries—for developing primary peritoneal cancer, a disease that begins in the lining, or peritoneum, of the abdomen.[4] The peritoneum cannot be removed during oophorectomy, and there's no proven method of preventing or screening for this rare cancer, which behaves like and is treated like stage 3 or 4 ovarian cancer.

BSO is not without side effects. It forever ends menstrual periods, which you may welcome, although it also ends fertility. If you don't plan to have children or you're already menopausal, oophorectomy might be an easy decision. It's not as straightforward if you want to pursue prophylactic BSO and also want to become pregnant. A fertility expert can explain your options, and your doctor can help you understand and manage your risk in the meantime. BSO also causes menopause. After surgery, medical intervention may be required to deal with mild to serious hot flashes, dry skin, vaginal dryness, and other symptoms. These symptoms (discussed in chapter 13) are less likely to occur in women who have BSO after natural menopause.

Oophorectomy Procedures

A surgeon needs clear access to the abdominal cavity to inspect the organs for cancer or other abnormalities before she removes the ovaries. She uses either of two techniques.

Laparoscopic BSO is frequently used to remove ovaries and tubes when cancer is not suspected. A tiny fiberoptic camera inserted through a small incision in the navel allows the surgeon to view the abdominal and pelvic areas on a video monitor. She makes two or three additional small incisions, through which she dissects and removes the ovaries. No sutures are required; only a small bandage covers the laparoscopic incision. The resulting scar is miniscule and eventually becomes almost invisible. Recovery after the one- to two-hour procedure may include an overnight hospital stay; some women go home the same day. Pain is controlled with medication during the first couple of weeks after surgery. Most women experience fatigue and need frequent rest throughout the day, recovering fully in one to two weeks.

Laparotomy, or abdominal oophorectomy, is performed when more access is needed to better view the abdomen. This might occur if you have scar tissue from previous surgeries, if your organs appear abnormal, or if the surgeon suspects cancer. In some cases, a laparoscopic oophorectomy ends up as a laparotomy if a larger incision is needed to control bleeding or a complication occurs. During laparotomy, a surgeon makes a four- to six-inch abdominal incision, cutting through the skin, fascia (connective tissue), and peritoneum. She cuts horizontally across the pubic hair line or vertically from the belly button down to the pubic bone. Although a horizontal scar is less noticeable, a vertical incision provides greater visibility into the abdomen and is always used when cancer is suspected. The surgeon pulls the abdominal muscles apart, inspects the organs, and removes the ovaries and fallopian tubes. When completed, she stitches the abdominal layers in reverse order and closes the incision with sutures or staples. A drain may be placed to collect excess fluid. Laparotomy takes about the same time as laparoscopy. Complications are more likely, and recovery is usually longer and more painful. Patients are discharged in two to five days. Abdominal discomfort and fatigue gradually subside after two weeks. Most exercise and lifting must wait until full recovery, usually in four to six weeks.

> ## EIGHT QUESTIONS FOR YOUR GYNECOLOGIC SURGEON
>
> 1. How many of these surgeries have you performed in high-risk women?
> 2. Do you recommend hysterectomy with oophorectomy?
> 3. What can I expect from these operations?
> 4. What are possible complications and how likely are they to occur?
> 5. How will you address these complications if they occur?
> 6. How long will I be in the hospital?
> 7. What should I expect and how should I prepare for recovery?
> 8. What long-term follow-up care will I need?

Either procedure should include an abdominal wash. This involves flushing sterile liquid into the pelvic cavity, removing the fluid, and sending it to a pathologist who looks for any evidence of cancer. If

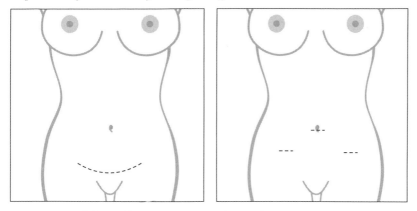

Laparotomy (*left*) and laparoscopic (*right*) oophorectomy incisions

you're at high risk, a *serial sectioning* of your ovaries and tubes is critically important.[5] This is a close pathological examination of several thin cross-sections of the fallopian tubes and ovaries to be certain no cancer is present. In some BRCA women, pathology reveals a small previously undetected cancer that requires chemotherapy and/or radiation treatment to prevent it from spreading.

Even though a gynecologist is trained to perform oophorectomy, it may be to your advantage to have your procedure done by a gynecologic oncologist, a specialist with advanced training who can also recognize and stage gynecologic cancers. If a gynecologist performs your oophorectomy and cancer is found, a second surgery may be needed to stage and determine the extent of the disease. Gynecologic oncologists, however, are familiar with the specific protocol for high-risk women, which includes exploring the pelvic organs for abnormalities or evidence of cancer, performing a peritoneal wash, and completely removing the ovaries and fallopian tubes. If cancer is found, she can remove lymph nodes and as much of the tumor as possible, and then treat you. The Society of Gynecologic Oncologists (www.sgo.org) will help you find a gynecologic oncologist.

Performed under general anesthesia in a hospital, BSO is a relatively safe operation, but it's still major surgery, and problems can occur (see table 13).

Table 13. Risks of gynecologic surgery

More common issues	Less common issues
Infection	Bleeding
Fluid or blood buildup at the surgical site (seroma/hematoma)	Blood loss
	Blood clots
Delayed healing	Long-term postoperative pain
	Intestinal blockage
	Injury to internal organs

EXPERT VIEW: Focus on the Fallopian Tubes

BY ELIZABETH SWISHER, M.D.

Oncologists have long assumed that ovarian carcinomas arise in the surface layer (epithelium) of the ovary or in the epithelial lining of small ovarian cysts. However, research suggests that so-called ovarian cancers may frequently originate in the fallopian tubes. The cancer may then implant and grow in the ovary and later be diagnosed as ovarian cancer. Several lines of evidence support this *tubal hypothesis*. Sometimes early BRCA cancers are found not in the ovary, but in the fallopian tubes during prophylactic surgery, and emerging data shows that even some sporadic ovarian cancers may begin in the fallopian tubes. Women whose ovaries are removed without also removing the fallopian tubes are at higher risk of later developing peritoneal cancer than those who have their tubes removed during ovarian surgery.

If the tubal hypothesis is correct, it will change how we diagnose ovarian cancer and possibly prevent it, since ultrasound imaging of the ovaries is not likely to be effective if the cancer begins somewhere else. At the University of Washington, we're studying high-definition endoscopy of the fallopian tubes: under anesthesia, we place a flexible, very thin endoscope into the fallopian tubes. If we can further refine this technology, one day we may be able to perform "falloposcopy" or visualization of the fallopian tubes as a screening method. Perhaps high-risk women who are not ready for BSO could have their fallopian tubes removed. The safety and efficacy involved aren't clear yet, but a better understanding of the origins of ovarian cancer will likely lead to improved prevention and early detection strategies.

Should You Have a Hysterectomy Too?

Hysterectomy, or removal of the uterus, is the second most common surgery (after cesarean delivery) among women in the United States. Most experts believe women with BRCA mutations have a uterine cancer risk that is similar to women in the general population. Therefore, hysterectomy isn't a standard recommendation with preventive BSO. You may want to have your uterus removed along with your ovaries and fallopian tubes if you:

- have had previous abnormal Pap smears, heavy bleeding, uterine fibroids, or other abnormalities of the uterus or cervix.
- have Lynch syndrome or other factors that increase your risk for uterine cancer.
- are concerned about increasing uterine cancer risk if you take tamoxifen.
- are considering hormones after surgery and prefer to take estrogen only, rather than a combination of estrogen and progesterone (discussed in chapter 13).
- are worried about your slight risk for developing cancer in the small fallopian tube remnant where it attaches to the uterus. Despite the fact that no cases of fallopian tube cancer in the remaining tissue have been reported, some gynecologic surgeons recommend hysterectomy with BSO to assure the tubes are entirely removed.

If you have a hysterectomy along with your oophorectomy, your ovaries, fallopian tubes, uterus, and usually your cervix will be removed in a single abdominal or laparoscopic procedure. If you have BSO with *laparoscopically assisted vaginal hysterectomy* (BSO/LAVH), your uterus and cervix will be removed through a vaginal incision. This entire procedure takes about two hours. Otherwise, you'll have a *total abdominal hysterectomy* with BSO (TAH/BSO), which involves the larger abdominal incision described earlier. TAH/BSO lasts two to four hours. Removing the uterus adds complexity to an oophorectomy, slightly increasing the potential for complications and requiring a lengthier recovery. You'll likely stay in the hospital overnight after BSO/LAVH and one or two nights after TAH/BSO.

You should also know:

- although *bladder prolapse*—the bladder sags down into the vagina—is cited as a risk with hysterectomy, it isn't common.
- reduced sexual satisfaction is sometimes mentioned as a possible side effect after hysterectomy, yet studies of women in the general population don't support this claim.
- the risk for operative infection is slightly increased if the uterus is removed during BSO.

Some surgeons perform BSO using a robotic system that produces 3-D abdominal images. This high-tech version of the laparoscopy provides a broader range of motion. Patients typically have less bleeding, fewer complications, and faster recovery. As with all surgeries, if you opt for robotic surgery, choose a surgeon who's experienced with this procedure. You might go home the same day or need to stay overnight in the hospital. Your scars will eventually fade and be barely visible.

MY STORY: Breaking the Family Curse

For as long as I can remember, the fear of breast cancer cast a shadow over my life. My grandmother died from it before I turned 5. When my mother was diagnosed at age 39, I viewed it as some kind of curse. My family was very secretive, and I felt alone with this. When my daughter was born, my joy was tempered by the thought that she would have breasts one day. Five years ago, when my aunt got ovarian cancer, a genetic counselor recommended my mother have testing. She carried a BRCA mutation; I later learned I had it too. I knew something was going on with the breast cancer in my family and felt sure I would not escape it, yet having it confirmed was devastating. I immediately had an oophorectomy. I was very, very angry about the gene. Having the mutation was beyond my control, and eventually knowing about it was a kind of blessing. —RANDI

Tubal Ligation

Normally performed for birth control, *tubal ligation* (tying your tubes) seals the fallopian tubes, preventing eggs from reaching the uterus. Some experts believe this may lower ovarian cancer risk for women who have a BRCA mutation. They don't recommend tubal ligation instead of oophorectomy to reduce risk, because it's unclear to what degree tubal ligation actually reduces the chance of developing cancer.

Oophorectomy, Mastectomy: Either, Neither, or Both?

If you have a BRCA mutation, you're concerned about managing your risk for both breast and ovarian cancer. Even without surgery, some women with a mutation will never get breast cancer, and most will never get ovarian cancer, making the decision to remove healthy organs more difficult.

Mastectomy is the most effective means of reducing breast cancer risk. Oophorectomy is the most effective way to lower ovarian cancer risk. Having both surgeries provides the greatest overall risk reduction. Which surgeries are right for you? Your personal circumstances and your tolerance for risk influence your decision about oophorectomy:

- You may be more reluctant to remove your ovaries if you're years away from menopause.

- If you're already experiencing symptoms from natural menopause, you may have fewer menopausal side effects from oophorectomy.
- You may want to delay surgery if you want to become pregnant at some point in the future.
- You may feel more anxious about your risk and more comfortable about oophorectomy if you have a family history of ovarian cancer.
- You may be more positive about surgery if you've had ovarian cysts, menstrual problems, or other gynecologic issues.

Some women opt to have both surgeries and be done with it. Others have one operation when they learn of their BRCA status and the other procedure later. As a 35-year-old woman who wants to have children, for example, you might have a prophylactic mastectomy right away, then have BSO after your children are born. Another woman of the same age might decide to have both mastectomy and BSO immediately to reduce her risk as much as possible, as soon as possible. Someone else may opt for increased surveillance with or without chemoprevention. If you find it difficult to decide whether you should have one surgery or the other, or both, consider the pros and cons in table 14.

Like mastectomy, oophorectomy and hysterectomy are irreversible operations and shouldn't be taken lightly. Deciding when to have oophorectomy to reduce your cancer risk is a personal choice, and one that should be made only after you've had time to research and thoughtfully consider all the ramifications of surgery. Genetics experts and gynecologic experts can help you sort out these issues, clarify different risk management options, and explain how each affects your risk. It's also helpful to speak with other high-risk women who have faced these same choices. Though they're not medical professionals, they offer a "been there, done that" sounding board for someone who is struggling with these perplexing decisions. The FORCE message boards are an excellent resource, where others at high risk share their experiences.

Table 14. Comparing mastectomy and gynecologic surgeries

	Benefits	*Limitations*
Mastectomy only	Reduces breast cancer risk	Loss of breasts; doesn't completely eliminate breast cancer risk; doesn't reduce ovarian cancer risk
BSO only	Reduces ovarian and breast cancer risk	Doesn't completely eliminate risk for peritoneal cancer; doesn't reduce breast cancer risk as much as mastectomy; routine screening for breast cancer is still required
	Eliminates menstrual periods	Causes menopause; eliminates ability to conceive (*in vitro* fertilization is still possible after oophorectomy if you keep your uterus)
Mastectomy combined with BSO	Provides maximum risk reduction for both breast and ovarian cancers	Doesn't completely eliminate risk for both; causes menopause and eliminates ability to conceive

Issues for Breast Cancer Survivors

If you've been diagnosed with breast cancer, other factors may influence your decision about oophorectomy and hysterectomy:

- If your cancer was estrogen or progesterone receptor–positive and you're still menstruating, oophorectomy may affect whether you're treated with aromatase inhibitors or tamoxifen.
- Oophorectomy may lower your risk of recurrence if you're premenopausal and your cancer was ER+ or PR+.

- If you had lumpectomy or unilateral mastectomy and still have breast tissue, oophorectomy lowers your risk for a new breast cancer diagnosis.

INSURANCE AND PAYMENT ISSUES

Some insurers consider payment based on individual circumstances; others still view prophylactic surgeries as elective and not medically necessary. As study data increasingly support the effectiveness of preventive oophorectomy, insurance companies are more likely to cover the surgery for high-risk individuals. Because surgery, recovery, and hospitalization are lengthier, some insurance companies won't pay for prophylactic hysterectomy unless you have a medical necessity. Review your insurance policy to determine whether a particular risk-reducing procedure is covered. If your request is denied, your physician and genetic counselor are your best defense. Ask them to provide letters of medical necessity on your behalf and assist with any appeals if coverage is denied.

THE FORCE PERSPECTIVE: DECIDING WHEN TO HAVE OOPHORECTOMY

Prophylactic BSO is recommended for all women who carry a BRCA mutation. Timing is an important consideration, because your ovarian cancer risk increases as you age. BSO is recommended between ages 35 and 40 and when childbearing is completed. (Although rare, ovarian cancers have been discovered in both BRCA1 and BRCA2 mutation carriers before age 35.) The younger you are when you have BSO, the greater your chance of avoiding ovarian cancer altogether. If you're a high-risk postmenopausal woman, experts recommend oophorectomy as soon as possible, because your risk is higher; your ovaries are producing few, if any, hormones; and side effects after BSO will likely be mild. As you think about when to have risk-reducing oophorectomy, consider these important factors:

- your current age and health status
- your risk for cancer now compared to your risk as you age

- your family planning choices
- risk-reducing benefits compared to menopausal symptoms and other side effects of surgery
- your schedule and lifestyle—you'll need sufficient time for surgery and recovery
- the lack of reliable screening tests for ovarian cancer
- your tolerance for living with greater risk if you decide to postpone oophorectomy (chemoprevention is also an option.)

WHAT TO REMEMBER ABOUT OOPHORECTOMY

- Oophorectomy cuts BRCA-related breast cancer risk by 50 percent.
- Prophylactically removing the fallopian tubes and ovaries is the standard of care for high-risk women. Both organs should be carefully examined in fine cross-section by a pathologist.
- A low risk for primary peritoneal cancer remains after BSO.
- Oophorectomy causes premature menopause (if you haven't reached natural menopause).

LEARN MORE ABOUT OOPHORECTOMY

The Foundation for Women's Cancer (www.foundationforwomens cancer.org or 312-578-1439) is organized by the Society of Gynecologic Oncologists. The foundation's mission is to support research, education, and public awareness of gynecologic cancer prevention, early detection, and optimal treatment.

Hystersisters (www.hystersisters.com) is a woman-to-woman support website for dealing with medical and emotional issues related to hysterectomy.

Ovarian Cancer Risk-Reducing Surgery: A Decision-Making Resource from the Fox Chase Cancer Center (www.fccc.edu/publications/ovarian -cancer-book.html) is available at no cost.

Chapter 13 Dealing with Menopause and Quality-of-Life Issues

OUR OVARIES PRODUCE about 90 percent of the estrogen, progesterone, and other reproductive hormones that keep our bones strong, provide some protection from heart disease, boost metabolism, and regulate the menstrual cycle. During our reproductive years, these hormones also increase sex drive, support pregnancy, and affect other critical body functions. For most women, menopause is a natural transition when the ovaries stop releasing eggs, menstrual periods cease, and our bodies make less estrogen and progesterone. Although other organs continue to produce small amounts, the overall level of circulating hormones is drastically decreased.

Women experience menopause on average at age 51. It can occur prematurely as a result of pelvic radiation, some gynecologic surgeries, certain chemotherapy, and some medications used to prevent or treat breast cancer. It may also occur for unknown reasons. Some women view menopause as a sorrowful ending to their youth, while others welcome its liberating aspects: no more menstrual cycles or worries about birth control. Young women who experience premature menopause after BSO may grieve the abrupt end to their fertility, yet even women in their fifties or older may experience a sense of grief and loss after surgery.

Symptoms of Surgical Menopause

Most women begin having symptoms a year or more before their periods end, as their estrogen levels gradually decline and fluctuate. This *perimenopause* may last a few years until menstruation stops completely, signaling the end of fertility. Having oophorectomy before natural menopause produces the same effect, bypassing the gradual transition of perimenopause and abruptly stopping hormone production—it can take days or weeks for most hormones to be removed from the body. Some women have no menopausal symptoms at all or find them to be only mildly distracting. For others, menopausal side effects are severe. Because surgical menopause is immediate, it sometimes causes symptoms that are more intense than those of a women experiencing natural menopause. If you're already menopausal when you have oophorectomy, you'll likely experience no change at all.

Hot Flashes

Hot flashes—episodes of mild to extreme heat throughout the body— are the most common side effect of menopause and are sometimes accompanied by heavy perspiration, a flushed face, or a rapid heartbeat. Your hot flashes may occur for just a short time after surgery, or they may come and go for years. They can be unpredictable and inopportune, occurring at work, in the car, or when you're with friends, so it's helpful to be prepared. Until they lessen—they eventually do—dress in layers. Notice whether spicy foods, alcohol, caffeine, or some activities trigger your hot flashes. Combat *night sweats* (hot flashes while you sleep) that can interrupt restful sleep by keeping your bedroom cool and well ventilated. Put a fan over your bed. Open the windows. (Partners or husbands can use an extra blanket or flannel bedclothes if they're cold.) Wear loose cotton bedclothes (or none at all) to promote circulation. Or tuck a Chillow, a soft, cooling pillow, into your pillowcase.

If anxiety appears to induce your hot flashes, try exercise, yoga, meditation, and other stress-management techniques. Some women say herbal supplements minimize their symptoms; no scientific data back this up. Despite Internet myth, *dong quai*, ginseng, black cohosh, and red clover haven't been proved effective either. Herbal preparations can be expensive, cause side effects, and may adversely interact with certain medications. Many contain concentrated amounts of plant estrogen, which may have the same effect as natural estrogen. Nor are herbal preparations regulated by the FDA; you don't know if you're getting the dosage or even the ingredients listed on the label.

Though vitamin E is often touted as a remedy for hot flashes, studies show it's ineffective, and it can slightly increase the risk for bleeding in certain women. Low-dose selective serotonin reuptake inhibitors (SSRIs), including the common antidepressants Paxil, Prozac, Effexor, and Lexapro, can lower the frequency and intensity of hot flashes in many women. They can also have side effects. They may reduce sex drive, and some (especially Paxil and Effexor) are associated with weight gain, so they may not be the best choice for all women. Some women find that exercise helps to reduce the frequency and intensity of hot flashes and helps promote deep and restful sleep. Estrogen replacement therapy (ERT) is the only medication specifically approved by the FDA for treating hot flashes.

Vaginal Dryness and Atrophy

The walls of the vagina are coated with a natural layer of moisture that increases and lubricates vaginal tissues when you're sexually aroused. After menopause, this moisture is secreted less frequently. Vaginal tissues may *atrophy*, or become thin and dry. In this condition, they can easily tear, bleed, or become infected. Atrophied tissue makes intercourse and even a Pap smear or vaginal exam painful. Douching can further dry the vagina. Frequent sexual stimulation will increase vaginal blood flow. Specially formulated over-the-counter vaginal lubricants make intercourse easier, and applying vaginal moisturizers or vitamin E oil relieves overly dry tissues. If your vaginal symptoms persist, ask your doctor about a prescription for a vaginal cream, tablet, or ring that releases small amounts of weak estrogen to the vaginal walls but minimizes absorption into the bloodstream. If you still have your uterus, ask your physician about progesterone creams that provide relief while protecting against uterine cancer risk.

Decreased Libido

Two hormones that affect a woman's sex drive, estrogen and testosterone, are significantly reduced after menopause. Many women continue to enjoy sexual intimacy. Others feel decreased sexual desire. Some physicians prescribe testosterone supplements to improve libido; it's unclear whether testosterone is as safe or even safer than estrogen. A small study found that bupropion (Wellbutrin) improved sexual arousal and satisfaction with intensity of orgasm when compared to placebo.[1] Another study showed that Wellbutrin increased satisfaction with sexual function among women who were treated with hormonal medications for breast cancer.[2] Neither research included women who had surgical menopause.

Changing certain lifestyle factors can often improve the situation. Suffering from hot flashes and feeling exhausted from lack of sleep can certainly diminish your libido. Worrying about your cancer risk, overall health, or other issues can also stifle sexual desire. You may need to change your approach to sex and intimacy to get the result you want. Good communication between you and your partner is essential, and making time for sex, finding new sources of arousal, and using methods other than intercourse are all possibilities. If all else fails, consider a visit to a sexual dysfunction expert.

Sleep Disturbances

Insomnia is a common complaint during menopause. It may be related to night sweats or other symptoms that disturb a good night's sleep. If you can't sleep through the night, especially if you have night sweats, you're better served by finding the cause of the problem rather than treating the symptoms. Avoid meals two or three hours before bedtime and cut down on or eliminate alcohol and caffeine. Exercise daily, but not within three hours of bedtime. Try to get to bed at the same time each night. Experts recommend that you read or do whatever makes you drowsy if you can't sleep after fifteen to twenty minutes. If you still need help to get a good night's rest, talk to your doctor about short-term medication, or consult with a sleep disorder clinic. Two unregulated supplements, valerian and kava, are popular sleep aids. Studies of valerian have produced inconclusive results; it does appear to improve sleep with few side effects if used in the short term. Kava can cause liver damage and should not be used.

Fatigue

Women frequently report feeling tired during menopause. If you're not getting adequate sleep, that may be the problem. A short nap during the day can help you recharge. Try not to sleep for more than an hour (just thirty minutes of napping can leave you refreshed) or after 3:00 p.m. Getting plenty of exercise, eating well, and tackling problems that interrupt your sleep should help you feel more energized. If you experience persistent fatigue, talk to your doctor about blood tests to rule out low thyroid or other conditions that may be the cause.

Mood Swings and Depression

It's not unusual to experience a range of feelings after oophorectomy. You may feel relieved because you've reduced your cancer risk, or sad and anxious about your long-term health, your remaining risk for cancer, or your loss of fertility. All these feelings are normal, and they're all okay, as long as negative emotions don't linger or interfere with your life. You may be happy one minute, and crying the next, for no apparent reason. St. John's wort may improve minor depression much like standard antidepressants do—study results have been inconsistent. But it may cause nausea, increase sensitivity to sun exposure, and interfere with aspirin, Coumadin, and other blood-thinning medications. Understanding why you feel the way you do is the first step to managing your emotional upheaval. A healthcare professional can help determine underlying physical causes of mood changes. If you feel severely depressed, it's very important to seek professional help. A mental healthcare professional can help you sort through your emotions and their causes and prescribe short-term medication if you need it.

Weight Gain

After menopause, changing hormones shift a woman's distribution of weight more to her abdomen; we tend to lose lean muscle, our metabolism slows, and we need fewer calories. The trick to avoiding weight gain during this time is ample exercise and a balanced reduced-calorie diet. Sounds simple, and it's nothing new, but the combination of diet and exercise is particularly important after menopause. This proven combination keeps weight in control; maintains bone, heart, and mental health; and reduces stress, hot flashes, and other symptoms of menopause and aging. Try for forty-five to sixty minutes of brisk walking or other weight-bearing aerobic exercise at least five days a week and resistance exercise three days a week to retain muscle mass and increase metabolism. Taking adequate amounts of calcium and vitamin D may also help keep the pounds off. When researchers followed more than thirty-six thousand participants in the Women's Health Initiative for seven years, they found that individuals who took 1,000 mg of calcium and 400 IU of vitamin D daily gained less weight than those who took a placebo.[3] If you're overweight, losing a few pounds can also decrease hot flashes.

GIVE YOGA A TRY

Some small studies show that yoga may improve hot flashes, mood swings, fatigue, joint pain, decreases in bone mineral density (weight-bearing yoga) associated with menopause, and overall quality of life. Even if yoga doesn't improve your symptoms, it improves flexibility and fitness and is worth adding to your exercise routine.

Sources: Carson JW, Carson KM, Porter LS, et al., "Yoga of Awareness Program for Menopausal Symptoms in Breast Cancer Survivors: Results from a Randomized Trial," *Supportive Care in Cancer* 17, no. 10 (2009): 1301–1309; Phoosuwan M, Kritpet T, Yuktanandana P, "The Effects of Weight-Bearing Yoga Training on the Bone Resorption Markers of Postmenopausal Women," *Journal of the Medical Association of Thailand* 92, Supplement 5 (2009): S102–S108; Tüzün S, Aktas I, Akarirmak U, et al., "Yoga Might Be an Alternative Training for the Quality of Life and Balance in Postmenopausal Osteoporosis," *European Journal of Physical Rehabilitation Medicine* 46, no.1 (2010): 69–72.

Skin and Hair Changes

Having less estrogen reduces collagen, and that can make hair and skin dry and thinner. You can greatly improve both by taking good care of your body. Drink water throughout the day to stay hydrated, avoid caffeine and alcoholic drinks, and eat enough fruits, vegetables, lean protein, and healthy fats, which help your skin from the inside. Facials and other skin care treatments can improve the appearance of your skin. Always use a strong sunblock when outdoors and moisturize throughout the day and before bed. Smoking decreases circulation and blood flow to the skin—yet another reason to quit.

Joint Pain

Some women develop achy, stiff, or painful joints after surgical menopause. Short-term over-the-counter anti-inflammatories like aspirin or NSAIDs can help. It's important to see your doctor to determine whether your pain is caused by arthritis. Ask about glucosamine, a supplement that relieves joint pain without serious side effects for some people. Your doctor may also suggest physical therapy or prescription medication.

Memory Changes

If you feel you're losing your mental edge after oophorectomy or you find it difficult to focus, there are several ways to improve the situation. First and foremost, start with your diet. Improve nutrition, avoid alcohol, and take a daily multivitamin. Exercise regularly and reduce stress. Engage your mind each day with reading, puzzles, or other brain-challenging activities. Sleep deprivation can also contribute to memory loss—get enough sleep and your memory may improve. Short-term hormone therapy might help after surgical menopause, which may be more detrimental to memory than natural menopause. Ginkgo biloba and other supplements are rumored to improve memory; none have proved effective.

Urinary Problems

Without estrogen, the *urethral sphincters* (muscles that control the flow of urine) thin and weaken, causing urinary incontinence (involuntary leaking of urine, which can further irritate already dry and thin vaginal tissue). After menopause, you may find you sometimes can't control your urine as well as before, and you may have a sudden urge to urinate when you laugh, cough, or sneeze. You can improve the condition by not smoking and by maintaining a healthy weight. You may be embarrassed to seek help for urinary incontinence, but it can often be greatly improved or completely cured. The first step is to see a doctor, who will perform a physical exam and analyze a sample of your urine. He may refer you to a urologist (a doctor who specializes in urinary conditions). In the meantime, absorbent pads can help avoid accidents, and pelvic floor exercises can strengthen your muscles and improve leaks. Other treatment options include electrical stimulation of the pelvic floor muscles, medications, surgery, and pelvic floor conditioning under the direction of healthcare professionals.

Long-Term Side Effects
Increased Risk for Heart Disease

Risk for heart disease, the leading cause of death in American women, increases after menopause, regardless of your age. The risk is higher if you have surgical menopause, because you have years ahead of you without the protective effects of natural estrogen. You may need medical intervention to combat later health issues. Heart disease includes *coronary artery disease*, when fatty deposits called *plaque* block arterial blood flow. If you smoke, you're at greater risk; stop smoking and your risk immediately drops. Other risk factors include a sedentary lifestyle, diabetes, a waistline of more than 35 inches, high blood pressure or cholesterol, and a family history of heart disease. A Mayo Clinic study of women who had surgical menopause before age 45 indicated that estrogen replacement therapy (ERT) may protect against heart disease associated with early menopause.[4] Hormone replacement therapy (HRT) did not provide similar protection. (A discussion of ERT and HRT follows later in this chapter.) If you have surgical menopause and don't take ERT, it's particularly important to exercise, monitor your cholesterol, try to maintain an ideal body weight, and consult with your doctors about reducing your risk for cardiovascular disease.

Bone Loss

Whether induced by nature or surgery, menopause accelerates bone loss, increasing the risk for fractures. Although some bone is lost naturally as we age, low levels of estrogen during menopause accelerates loss—nearly 1 in 4 people who have hip fractures after age 50 die within a year, usually from pneumonia that develops from lack of mobility.[5] Healthcare professionals often recommend a baseline bone density test with *dual-energy x-ray absorptiometry* (DEXA) to measure the calcium and mineral content of the hip and spine before prophylactic oophorectomy or soon after, with a follow-up every year or two after menopause. DEXA results are categorized as normal, *osteopenia*, or osteoporosis. Normal thinning means bone density is about the same as other women your age. Osteopenia refers to bone mass below normal levels compared to women your age. This isn't a medical condition; it's simply a method of categorizing individuals who may be at risk for more serious bone thinning. If osteopenia is a concern, your doctor will discuss ways to strengthen your bones and prevent or slow further bone loss. Options include bone-building medications, a weight-bearing exercise regimen, and taking calcium and vitamin D supplements.

Left untreated, osteopenia can lead to osteoporosis, a serious condition that develops when bones are brittle and weak, lose more mineral density than your body can replace, and may easily break. Osteoporosis medication may have side effects, and some may raise the risk for other cancers. If you have menopause-related osteopenia or osteoporosis, consult with an endocrinologist or other healthcare professional who is trained in managing menopausal symptoms. Osteoporosis treatments include the following:

- Bisphosphonates, including Actonel, Boniva, Fosamax, and Reclast, preserve bone density. These drugs can cause nausea, heartburn, and pain in the arms and legs. If you have unacceptable side effects with one brand, you might do well with another. A clinical trial is trying to determine whether zoledronic acid (Zometa), an injectable bisphosphonate, reduces bone loss after risk-reducing oophorectomy. (For study updates, visit clinicaltrials. gov and type in "GOG 0215.") In very rare cases, bisphosphonates can cause *osteonecrosis* of the jaw, an infection that develops when the bone doesn't get enough blood and begins to deteriorate. When identified early, osteonecrosis is treated with antibiotics; surgery may be required, depending on the extent of bone loss. Bisphosphonates may also increase esophageal cancer risk.

> **SEVEN STEPS TO BETTER BONE HEALTH**
>
> 1. Don't smoke.
> 2. Avoid or limit alcoholic beverages.
> 3. Limit intake of cola drinks.
> 4. Get at least 1,200 mg of calcium through diet and supplementation.
> 5. Get the daily recommended amount of vitamin D for your age.
> 6. Determine whether the medications you take affect bone loss.
> 7. Perform weight-bearing or resistance exercise for at least thirty minutes a day, three days a week.

- Raloxifene is approved by the FDA to prevent and treat osteoporosis.
- Low-dose, short-term ERT or HRT prevents and treats osteoporosis (see "Should You Take Hormones?" in this chapter).
- Calcitonin mimics a natural hormone that can improve bone strength. Taken by injection or nasal spray, it's prescribed for women who have been menopausal for at least five years. Aside from mild nasal irritation, it appears to be without serious side effects.
- Parathyroid hormone (PTH), which involves expensive daily injections, creates new bone. Used for 18 to 24 months, PTH doesn't protect against bone loss once women stop using it. Teriparatide (Forteo) is a synthetic form of PTH for women with very low bone density.

Should You Take Hormones?

The question on most women's minds after oophorectomy is "Should I take hormones to combat my menopausal symptoms?" quickly followed by "Are they safe?" It may seem contrary for high-risk women to take hormones after preventive oophorectomy. However, the net effect is usually a lower level of hormones than you had before the surgery. Research suggests that short-term use of hormones doesn't increase breast cancer risk in previvors who have BRCA mutations and experience surgical menopause from BSO.[6] Additional studies with longer follow-up are needed to confirm the long-term safety of hormones.

The menopause experience is different for every woman. Finding just the right remedy is often a trial-and-error process. Low-dose hormone pills, creams, lotions, gels, vaginal rings, or patches are options to address persisting symptoms that affect your quality of life. Even if you don't experience symptoms, talk to your doctor about whether the overall benefits of hormones outweigh the risks for you. Two types of hormone therapies treat postmenopausal symptoms after natural or surgical menopause—each has benefits and risks.

After hysterectomy, ERT is often prescribed for women who no longer have a uterus. The most common ERT is conjugated estrogen tablets (Premarin) made from pregnant horse urine. ERT is linked with gall bladder disease and may increase risk for blood clots, particularly in women who smoke or take oral estrogen; the risk is not as high if you use a low-dose estrogen skin patch instead. ERT also slightly increases the risk for uterine cancer, and if you still have your ovaries, ERT and HRT may raise ovarian cancer risk. If you still have your uterus, synthetic progesterone combined with estrogen (HRT) protects against uterine cancer. HRT has the same possible side effects as ERT and may elevate breast cancer risk in women who have natural menopause.

This is all confusing, and it's difficult to know which hormone therapy, if any, is right for you. Health experts consider limited hormone use appropriate for the high-risk population, given the following:

- After BSO, women with BRCA mutations decrease (but don't entirely erase) their breast cancer risk. Studies show that when these women took HRT or ERT, their risk remained lower for the three-and-a-half-year follow-up period after surgery.[7] Longer studies are needed to determine whether risk reduction persists beyond that period.

- Hormones may be safer for previvors after PBM (they have very little breast tissue) and BSO.

- ERT alone doesn't appear to significantly increase breast cancer risk in the general population.[8]

EXPERT VIEW: What We Learned from the Women's Health Initiative

CAROL J. FABIAN, M.D.

Few issues cause as much angst as whether or not to take hormone replacement therapy. To determine whether taking hormones was beneficial in improving overall health and reducing deaths, the randomized, placebo-controlled trials in the Women's Health Initiative (WHI) were launched for women 50 or older. Oral estrogen combined with progestin was used for women with a uterus; estrogen alone was used for women without a uterus. Unlike the real-world scenario in which women usually start hormones in their late 40s and early 50s, and take them for an average of three years, participants who started hormones were 63 on average.

Although women on HRT had fewer colon cancers and bone fractures, they had more breast cancers, blood clots, stroke, and heart attacks. Most of these adverse events occurred in women in their 60s and 70s. Women in the ERT group did not appear to have an increased risk for breast cancer, and those starting oral ERT in their 50s or within ten years of menopause had fewer cardiovascular events. This suggests a health advantage to avoiding oral progestins. Some young, high-risk women contemplating preventive removal of their ovaries and tubes might consider removing their uterus so that they can take ERT without increasing risk for uterine cancer. Women who want to keep their uterus should speak with their doctor about ways to minimize their progestin dose.

Bioidenticals, Compounded Hormones, and Other Alternatives

Bioidenticals are hormones derived from animal, plant, or synthetic sources that are chemically identical to the hormones made by the body. No evidence shows that bioidenticals are safer or more effective than commercial hormone preparations. Both are approved by the FDA and are available by prescription to treat menopause symptoms.

Companies aggressively market supplements and herbal concoctions, often with misleading advertisements. Although the hype is appealing, and increasing numbers of women are using unapproved hormones to decrease hot flashes and other symptoms, they may also be taking risks with their health. Because these products are classified as supplements, they're untested, unapproved, and unregulated by the FDA. No research supports manufacturers' claims that their products are more natural, safer alternatives to FDA-approved hormonal medications or proves that these products are safe, that they are consistently prepared, or that they even work. Many are sold as cure-all menopausal fountains of youth. Some contain phytoestrogens. Others contain estriol, an estrogen that occurs during a woman's pregnancy and may increase breast cancer risk. Estriol hasn't been studied sufficiently to prove it's a safe or effective antidote for menopausal symptoms.

Some physicians prefer to prescribe *compounded* (custom-mixed) hormones and consider them to be safer or more effective than commercial HRT. Little research compares them to commercial hormone preparations. Compounded hormones may have risks—they're neither tested nor approved by the FDA. They're also unregulated, so preparations may vary between pharmacists and from one prescription to the next. When the FDA analyzed twenty-nine such products in 2001, ten samples (34 percent) failed quality tests; nine of the products contained less of the active ingredient than listed on the label.[9] In 2008, the agency warned seven compounding pharmacies that their products were unsupported by medical evidence and were considered false and misleading. The North American Menopause Society (NAMS) doesn't recommend custom-compounded products over well-tested, government-approved products for most women. Nor does it recommend saliva testing to determine a woman's hormone levels, a common practice by physicians who prescribe compounded preparations.

MY STORY: I Have to Do What's Right for Me

*As a previvor with a BRCA1 mutation, I had BSO at age 39. I began having hot flashes and night sweats, but they were bearable. I decided not to use HRT; then six months after my surgery, I started vaginal estrogen for severe vaginal atrophy. A bone scan showed I also had osteopenia; a second scan the following year showed I was losing bone. I preferred to try to increase my bone mass with diet and exercise instead of taking a bisphosphonate. After doing my own research on the safety and benefits of hormones on bone and cardiovascular health and menopausal symptoms, I decided to begin HRT more for my long-term health than my hot flashes and night sweats. After two years of using a combined estrogen-progesterone patch and vaginal estrogen, my bone mass increased. I'm young and active, and I want to stay that way. I'm not sure whether HRT or diet and exercise (or both) are responsible. I'm protecting my health the best way I can. —*EVA*

Issues for Breast Cancer Survivors

If you've had ER+ breast cancer, the risks of taking hormones may outweigh the benefits. The HABITS trial in 2004 verified that HRT (not ERT) increases the risk of local recurrence and a second breast cancer in women who had remaining breast tissue.[10] Other studies have found no difference in recurrence rates. Some doctors allow patients to try vaginal estrogen. In situations where no other remedy restores a woman's quality of life, women may choose low-dose hormones after thoroughly considering the benefits and risks. If you're a survivor struggling with the symptoms of menopause, talk with your healthcare team about the remedies described in this chapter. If your symptoms persist, ask your doctor for a referral to an endocrinologist who has expertise in menopause.

INSURANCE AND PAYMENT ISSUES

Not all insurance policies pay for bone density checks, hormone therapy based on saliva tests, or custom-compounded preparations, so check with your carrier to determine whether you're covered.

THE FORCE PERSPECTIVE: MENOPAUSE IS PERSONAL

Deciding whether HRT is right for you is a personal decision that can frustrate and confuse. Don't automatically assume you need hormones. If you prefer to avoid them, see how you fare following oophorectomy. If lifestyle changes and nonhormonal treatments don't adequately manage your menopause symptoms, speak with your doctor about treatment options, considering your risk status. Perception can make a big difference. In controlled studies, women who took placebos but believed them to be medication reported improved hot flashes 40 percent of the time. Try not to be influenced by other people's perception of what menopause is supposed to be like, and let your own experience determine whether you need ERT or HRT. Women often say their fear of surgical menopause without hormones keeps them from oophorectomy. Afraid of accelerated aging from BSO before menopause, they also fear increasing cancer risk if they take hormones. Many experts believe hormone replacement after oophorectomy is safe for previvors, and the amount of hormones you take will be less than what your ovaries produced on their own.

WHAT TO REMEMBER ABOUT MENOPAUSE

- Menopause symptoms may be mild, severe, or nonexistent.
- Symptoms may be more intense after risk-reducing oophorectomy than in natural menopause. Exercising can help reduce the severity of symptoms.
- Some symptoms are well tolerated with over-the-counter aids or nonmedical interventions. More persistent symptoms may require prescription medications or hormone preparations.

- Discuss the risk and benefits of hormone replacement with your healthcare team before deciding if they're for you.

LEARN MORE ABOUT MENOPAUSE

The North American Menopause Society (www.menopause.org) is devoted to promoting women's health and quality of life through an understanding of menopause.

I'm Not in the Mood: What Every Woman Should Know about Improving Her Libido, by Judith Reichman, explores medical reasons for loss of libido.

Restore Yourself: A Woman's Guide to Reviving Her Sexual Desire and Passion for Life, by James A. Simon, M.D., and Victoria Houston, provides helpful information for women who suffer from diminished sex drive after menopause.

PART FOUR LIVING WITH BRCA

Issues and Answers

Chapter 14 Managing Lifestyle

Choices

WE CAN'T NEGATE THE FACT THAT AGE, inherited predisposition, and other factors beyond our control increase cancer risk. But cancers don't develop overnight. *Carcinogenesis*, the multistep evolution from normal cell to cancer, usually takes several years, providing opportunity (especially the younger we are) to potentially offset inherited risk with intervening behaviors. Being genetically predisposed doesn't necessarily mean you're destined to develop cancer unless something in your lifestyle, environment, or the aging process creates irreparable damage that prompts damaged cells to replicate out of control and form tumors.

We don't have enough large well-controlled studies to know exactly what causes breast or ovarian cancer in people of average or high risk, or exactly how lifestyle and environmental factors influence risk. One research project—or ten or twenty—doesn't necessarily produce unequivocal results. Studies conducted in different ways with different controls often reach conclusions that don't necessarily prove cause and effect. An observational study of more than thirty-five thousand postmenopausal women, for example, suggested those who regularly used fish oil supplements were less likely to develop breast cancer over the next six years.[1] However, the study didn't look at other influencing factors.

Health experts can't recommend one behavior or another until clinical trials prove it beneficially affects human cancer risk or at the very least won't cause harm. Even laboratory tests that produce results in rats are just a step in the process. That's why trying to act on every research report in the news—"soy protects against breast cancer risk," or "soy increases breast cancer risk"—can make you crazy. Although scientists haven't yet discovered many controllable factors that affect cancer risk, we can focus on four that are well studied: nutrition, weight, physical activity, and alcohol consumption.

The Three-Legged Stool: Nutrition, Weight, and Physical Activity

Most confirmed data about the effect of lifestyle behaviors on the risk for disease, including breast and ovarian cancer, can be summed up in just three words: nutrition, weight, and exercise. Combined, these closely related risk factors are like the three legs of a stool. Control all three and you have a balanced approach to limiting cellular damage that can progress to disease. Allow any one element to get out of whack, and your risk may tip in favor of cancer.

Nutrition

While a direct link between most individual foods and cancer hasn't been made, the indirect relationship is clear: your body needs essential nutrients to function optimally, with a strong immune system that can better repair genetic damage before cancer occurs. Managing what you eat to control your weight is also important, because being overweight increases the likelihood of developing heart disease, diabetes, and cancer.

Cancer was less prevalent during your grandparents' time. It's probably no coincidence that they were more active than you are and ate a more nutritious diet than you do today. Eating habits and food sources were very different forty or fifty years ago, with little or no fast food. Our rate of cancer is much higher than the rate in Africa, Asia, and other cultures where fruits, vegetables, and whole grains account for 50 to 90 percent of the average diet. A consistent diet of foods with hormones, transfats, processed sweeteners, and artificial fillers may cause DNA changes that can lead to cancer. If our children follow the same damaging lifestyle patterns, they'll continue the cycle of damage and disease. In fact, what you eat may affect your children and grandchildren's risk for cancer, regardless of their diet. Georgetown University Medical Center researchers showed that rats who ate a fatty, unhealthy diet passed on DNA damage and increased breast cancer risk to their daughters and granddaughters; half the grandchildren developed breast tumors, even though they ate a normal diet. When both grandmother rats ate fatty diets, 80 percent of subsequent grandchildren developed tumors.[2] This may partially explain why certain cancers run in some families, even in the absence of a specific genetic mutation.

The exact effect of diet and its impact on hereditary cancer risk is still unclear. A high-fat diet is known to increase heart disease, blood pressure, and many other health problems—at least one study linked a high-fat diet during adolescence with increased premenopausal breast cancer risk—yet it hasn't been proved to increase cancer risk.[3] Although evidence doesn't decisively show that a diet high in vegetables reduces breast and ovarian cancer risk, research increasingly emphasizes the value of plant-based foods. Low-calorie, high-fiber produce contains more than fifty-five nutrients and *phytochemicals*, which have *antioxidant* properties that protect cells and help repair DNA damage. Cruciferous vegetables (broccoli, Brussels sprouts, cauliflower); orange, red, and purple fruits and vegetables; tea; and red wine are rich in both nutrients and phytochemicals. The American Institute for Cancer Research recommends meals that are two-thirds or more fruits, vegetables, beans, and whole grains, and one-third or less lean protein.

Are Some Foods Protective?

It's very difficult to study how diet affects cancer risk over a lifetime, because researchers can't control the long-term diets of study participants, and when questioned, people often don't accurately recall what they've eaten over many years. Even though breast cancer has been studied more than ovarian cancer, including relationships between diet and risk, results are often inconsistent. Many foods, including green tea, garlic, mushrooms, avocados, and others (see chapter 17 for specific information about pomegranate for prostate cancer), contain beneficial nutrients and phytochemicals. None is proved to prevent cancer. Genes affect how our bodies metabolize and use medications like tamoxifen; it's likely they also affect how we metabolize food. Scientists won't be able to predict how particular foods affect breast or ovarian cancer, and specifically hereditary risk, until they're able to isolate and understand harmful or beneficial compounds in various foods and explain how genetically different individuals metabolize them. For now, experts recommend balanced meals that include a variety of nutritious foods. An observational study of women with BRCA mutations found lower breast cancer risk in those who had varied diets.[4]

The link between dietary soy and breast cancer risk has been studied extensively, producing inconclusive results. Women in the United States are more likely to develop and die from breast cancer than women throughout Asia, where the population consumes less fat and where soy is a staple. When Asian women move to the United States and assume our lifestyle, their breast cancer rates rise, becoming similar to ours in a few generations. Researchers theorize that the Asian high-soy diet might be the protective factor, yet studies haven't consistently proved that soy is responsible for the reduced risk. No specific research has examined the direct effect of soy on BRCA-related cancer risk.

Soy has been studied extensively, with conflicting results. Along with many other legumes and vegetables, it contains high levels of *phytoestrogens*, plant-based estrogens that may act like tamoxifen and block the effects of estrogen on breast tissue. On the flip side, phytoestrogen may also act like weak estrogen, and some oncologists recommend women with ER+ cancers avoid it altogether. Soy is a complete source of protein for vegetarians, however, and most experts consider eating it three times a week to be safe, even for survivors. Because the long-term safety of consuming highly concentrated soy phytoestrogens is unknown, soy supplements and beverages or food products containing concentrated soy additives should be avoided. Some studies link diets high in phytoestrogens to reduced breast cancer risk; others show it may not have a significant effect. When researchers analyzed twenty-one studies of *lignans*—a type of phytoestrogen in many fruits, vegetables, and whole grains—they found that postmenopausal women who ate lignan-rich foods were 14 percent less likely to develop breast cancer than those with low intakes.[5] (Flaxseed is the best food source of lignans.) Premenopausal women didn't have the same reduced risk, and the study didn't specifically address women with BRCA mutations.

Numerous large studies in various countries consistently show no link between midlife intake of dairy and increased breast cancer risk. What you eat during adolescence and young adulthood, however, may affect your risk later in life. Dairy products in young adulthood may lower the risk for breast cancer, but some evidence suggests high-fat dairy such as butter may be detrimental.[6] Nonfat dairy is safer, if not beneficial, compared to high-fat dairy products. Whole milk is appropriate for toddlers or people who have trouble getting the fat and calories they need. It's not the best choice for most adults. One cup of whole milk has 150 calories and 8 grams of fat. Low-fat milk is better, although it still has 120 calories and 5 grams of fat. Nonfat (skim) milk has the same amount of protein and calcium, with just 80 calories and less than 1 gram per serving of fat.

> **A GUIDE TO THE SMART PANTRY**
>
> - lean proteins (skinless poultry, seafood, beans, and nonfat dairy products)
> - healthy fats (walnuts; flax; fatty fish; olive, peanut, and canola oils)
> - whole grains (whole grain cereals, breads, brown rice, and pasta)
> - nuts and seeds (almond, Brazil, pumpkin, sunflower, and sesame)
> - a colorful variety of fresh or frozen fruits and vegetables
> - limited red meats, salt, sugar, butter, and transfats; products made with refined white flour; and fast or processed foods

Supplements

Despite what you may have heard or read, little clinical evidence supports the premise that supplements reduce cancer risk, and high doses of some supplements may actually increase cancer risk. Promising research is under way, yet experts can't recommend specific quantities of selenium, lycopene, caffeine, or various supplements and antioxidants to lower cancer risk. Having sufficient levels of vitamin D is important because, aside from helping the body absorb calcium, it reduces inflammation and modulates the immune system. Although salmon and sardines are good sources, as are fortified milk and cereals, most vitamin D is made in the body when skin is exposed to sunlight—just fifteen minutes per day is sufficient. Although several observational studies indicate vitamin D may be helpful against breast and colon cancer, research results on its effect on prostate and pancreatic cancer risk have been mixed. Clinical trials are under way to evaluate the effects of vitamin D in high-risk women. Researchers are also studying whether *diindolymethane* (DIM), a natural compound found in cruciferous vegetables, may lower breast cancer risk in BRCA mutation carriers.

Fish oil, another component of Asian diets, is a rich source of omega-3 fatty acids. It may lower breast cancer risk in the general population; no studies have reviewed the oil's effect in women with BRCA mutations. In an observational study of thirty-five thousand postmenopausal women, those who said they regularly used fish oil supplements were one-third less likely to develop breast cancer over the next six years than nonusers.[7] Researchers are investigating whether fish oil and vitamin supplements affect breast cancer and prostate cancer risks. Salmon, tuna, sardines, trout, and mackerel are good sources of omega-3. Some have high levels of mercury, so limit consumption to two or three servings a week of wild-caught fish. Farmed salmon tends to have more contaminants and less omega-3. For many people, fish oil capsules are more readily available and convenient. Walnuts, flaxseeds, sesame seeds, and certain vegetables have oils that include *alpha-linolenic acid*, a molecule that our bodies can convert to omega-3 fatty acids.

Too Much of the Good Life: Controlling Your Weight

You've heard it time and again, and it bears repeating: your weight matters. Two-thirds of Americans over age 20 are overweight, and one-third are obese, increasing their odds of many health conditions, including breast cancer. We eat too many of the wrong things and simply eat too much. Obesity has doubled among adults in the last twenty years and more than tripled among adolescents in that time.[8] According to the American Institute for Cancer Research, poor diet, physical inactivity, and excess body fat cause one-third of all cancers, including postmenopausal breast cancer, among Americans.[9] That's bad news for us, and it's worse for our children, who may be the first generation in U.S. history to have shorter life expectancies than their parents because of excess weight. Some of the strongest evidence shows that excess fat increases estrogen levels. It may also reduce immune function and raise cellular stress that can cause DNA damage. American Cancer Society research found a higher rate of death from ovarian cancer in obese women; the heaviest women had a 50 percent greater risk.[10]

If you need to lose weight, don't waste your time on fad diets that generally disregard the rudimentary rule of weight control—calories in, calories out. While you may lose pounds in the interim, the weight usually returns when your diet ends. To maintain a healthy weight, make better choices in the grocery store. Follow a sensible long-term strategy: exercise and eat right to gradually shed weight, and maintain an exercise and eating regimen that keeps you satisfied and fit without dieting.

When HRT was found to increase cancer risk in postmenopausal women of average risk, millions of women stopped cold turkey, reducing

CALCULATING OBESITY AND WAIST CIRCUMFERENCE

You're considered overweight if your body mass index (BMI) is 25.0 to 29.9. You're considered obese and at higher risk for several diseases, including breast cancer, if your BMI is 30.0 or greater. Use the calculator at What Health (www.whathealth.com/bmi/calculator.html), or calculate your own BMI: 703 x weight in pounds ÷ (height in inches)^2. A woman who weighs 170 pounds and is 5' 5" tall has a BMI of 28 (119,510 ÷ 4,225). Waist circumference is also an important measurement. According to the United States Department of Health and Human Services, women with a waist circumference of more than 35 inches are at increased risk for developing chronic diseases. (The McKinley Health Center provides a handout about how to measure your waist: www.mckinley.illinois.edu/handouts/waist_circumference/waist_circumference.htm.)

the overall rate of sporadic breast cancers. That's an example of how changing a lifestyle factor can influence cancer risk. The International Agency for Research on Cancer says the same thing would happen if more women lost weight and exercised more. Losing even 10 to 15 pounds positively impacts this risk. If you have a BRCA mutation, it's particularly important to stay as lean as possible throughout your life. Analysis of women with BRCA mutations showed that those with normal weight at menarche and lighter weight at age 21 had delayed onset of breast cancer.[11] In a five-country study involving 1,073 women, those with BRCA1 mutations reduced their breast cancer risk when they lost as little as 10 pounds between ages 18 and 30.[12]

Physical Activity

Staying active throughout your life strengthens your heart and cardiovascular system, prevents obesity, modulates hormone levels, and lowers risks in unexplained ways. Combined with a sensible caloric intake, it's the most effective way to avoid excess pounds and maintain a lifelong healthy weight. A study of women with BRCA mutations showed that those who were active in sports, dance, or casual exercise during their teen years delayed the onset of breast cancer later in life.[13] After age 25, women tend to add a few pounds each year, even if they don't eat more, due to reduced activity and loss of muscle. With less muscle, your

---

SEVEN WAYS TO LOSE WEIGHT AND KEEP IT OFF

1. Adopt a physically active lifestyle to maintain your ideal weight.
2. Find exercises you enjoy—dance, hike, swim, or do Pilates—and change your regimen frequently.
3. Exercise each day. The American Institute for Cancer Research recommends starting with thirty minutes of moderate daily activity, gradually building to thirty minutes of vigorous exercise (you should sweat) or sixty minutes of moderate exercise daily.
4. Strength train two to three times weekly to improve bone strength and rev up your metabolism.
5. Incorporate more exercise into your normal routine. Walk to lunch instead of driving or use the treadmill as you watch TV.
6. Set gradual weight loss goals (lose 1 to 2 pounds per week) instead of one big one (lose 60 pounds).
7. Make a commitment to fitness. Momentum is a powerful force.

metabolism (rate of burning calories) slows. It's difficult to lose weight through exercise alone, and the more you eat, the more calories you must burn to lose weight or maintain a healthy weight. (It takes sixty-nine minutes to lose just 300 calories if you walk at twenty minutes per mile.) It's never too late to transform poor nutrition and sedentary habits into a healthy, fit lifestyle. Always discuss any new exercise program with your physician, especially if you're in treatment, recovering from surgery, or at risk for lymphedema.

EXPERT VIEW: Integrative Medicine and Hereditary Cancer

BY DILJEET K. SINGH, M.D., PH.D.

Women with inherited predisposition to breast and ovarian cancer can benefit substantially from integrative medicine and oncology. *Nutrigenomics* (how diet affects gene expression) and *epigenetics* (inherited modifications of gene expression) show that what we eat and how we live can influence how our genes behave. Integrative oncology focuses on the innate healing abilities of our bodies and the tools we have to support these abilities. Integrative medicine includes biologically based practices (diet, dietary supplements, herbs), mind-body medicine (guided imagery, hypnosis, meditation, stress management, social support), manipulative, or body-based, practices (massage therapy, reflexology), energy medicine (acupuncture, Qigong, Reiki, yoga), and whole system approaches (Ayurveda, traditional Chinese medicine, homeopathy). Although no studies of lifestyle modification specifically focus on BRCA mutation carriers, data from other populations tell us that lifestyle, including diet, exercise, and stress management, has a tremendous impact on our likelihood of developing cancer. Adherence to a healthy diet, regular physical activity, and individualized approaches to stress management are the first essential steps in an integrative approach to optimal health for high-risk women.

MY STORY: I Did Everything Right and Still Got Breast Cancer

At 33, I was shocked to be diagnosed with breast cancer. I didn't drink or smoke. I had been a vegetarian for almost ten years, and had exercised and

(continued)

followed recommendations for protecting myself. I breastfed my baby for over six months. My diagnosis made more sense when I later learned I had a mutation; my genes were a stronger influence than my lifestyle. Although I lived a healthy lifestyle as an adult, as a teen I drank, smoked, and ate high-fat fast foods. I was overweight then and didn't exercise much. If I had known about my genetic destiny at age 16, I like to think I would have made better choices about my health. I'll never know for sure, but I believe my healthy lifestyle as an adult may have saved me from a worse prognosis. It certainly helped me get through treatment with fewer side effects. You're never too young to live a healthy life. —SUSANNE

Alcohol: An Unwise Choice

There's no longer a question whether alcohol increases breast cancer risk in the general population—it does. Moderate alcohol appears to be heart healthy, but it also increases blood estrogen levels, and that raises breast cancer risk. How much is too much? Most research points to increased risk with just one or two drinks per day. (One drink is 12 ounces of beer, 5 ounces of wine, or 1½ ounces of 80-proof spirits.) The more you drink, the higher your risk, and all forms of alcohol damage cells. Routine drinking is the problem—a glass or two of beer or wine occasionally isn't going to make a difference. According to the American Cancer Society, women who regularly have even a few drinks per week, especially those who don't get enough folate, raise their breast cancer risk. The equivalent of 4 ounces (½ cup) a day slightly raises risk in the general population; that risk increases more significantly after menopause. It's unclear whether previvors with BRCA mutations are affected in the same way.

Other Lifestyle Risk Factors
Hormone Replacement

For many high-risk women, replacement hormones provide welcome relief from menopausal symptoms. Most large studies on hormone replacement therapy included women with average cancer risk who took hormones after natural menopause. In this population, HRT (estrogen plus progesterone) increased breast cancer risk when used for more than five years. ERT (estrogen alone) did not. The research on HRT is somewhat more reassuring for previvors with BRCA mutations who have BSO before menopause: short-term (up to three years), low-dose HRT appears to be safe and doesn't increase the risk for breast cancer.[14] After natural menopause, both ERT and HRT may raise ovarian cancer risk in women with average risk.

When experts examined the health records of nearly 1 million Danish women, they discovered a 38 percent higher risk of ovarian cancer among those taking traditional or bioidentical hormones, regardless of dose, length of time used, or whether they took ERT or HRT.[15] While the risks of short-term HRT are minimal for previvors after PBM and BSO, it isn't recommended for postmenopausal mutation carriers who still have their breasts and ovaries. Whether to use hormones is an individual decision and requires discussion with healthcare providers who have expertise in hereditary cancer and menopause.

Smoking

If you smoke, do whatever you must to quit. It damages your heart and lungs and is detrimental to your health on many levels. An analysis of several studies shows that women in the general population who begin smoking at an early age and premenopausal women who are exposed to secondhand smoke have higher rates of breast cancer than women who never smoke.[16] After diagnosis, smoking also increases the odds of a new tumor in the opposite breast.[17] In the general population, smoking also raises risk for cancer in several organs, including the ovaries, pancreas, bladder, lungs, kidneys, and throat. If you're a smoker and you develop cancer, smoking can interfere with treatment, promote infection, and delay healing. It may also delay surgery, including breast reconstruction; you'll need to quit for several weeks before and after. Ask your doctor about medications that can help you quit or use the

American Lung Association's smoking-cessation program (www.lung usa.org).

Environmental Exposure

Life in the twenty-first century involves exposure to innumerable pollutants, pesticides, and chemicals. (Take a look at your inventory of everyday products: are *any* of them chemical-free?) High-dose exposure to many of these substances produce breast tumors in lab animals. Whether the same is true in humans, specifically high-risk women or women with BRCA mutations, remains unclear. If you have a BRCA mutation, you may be particularly sensitive to environmental toxins that may cause genetic damage. Having a BRCA2 mutation makes you more susceptible to melanoma, for example, so you would need to take extra precautions to protect yourself from harmful sun exposure, including wearing sunblock and sun-protective clothing when outdoors.

Cumulative radiation exposure promotes genetic damage and formation of cancerous cells. Chest radiation as a child or young adult, for example, elevates your risk of developing breast cancer later in life. Current breast radiation therapy delivers a much lower dose. Radiation from yearly mammograms may affect the risk for cell damage, particularly before age 30; experts believe the benefits of routine mammography outweigh its limited exposure. Consider using a digital mammogram facility, if available. CT scans or other diagnostic tests that expose you to radiation should be performed only when medically necessary.

Several studies associate nighttime exposure to artificial light with increased rates of breast cancer. The exposure reduces production of *melatonin*, a hormone that may lower cancer risk. Female nurses and other women who work night shifts have higher rates of breast cancer—rates are lower among the blind and women in underdeveloped countries, where artificial lighting is less common. The International Agency for Research on Cancer, a branch of the World Health Organization, already classifies night-shift work as a "probable carcinogen."

You may have heard about two other widely used chemicals that potentially affect breast cancer risk. Small amounts of *bisphenol A* (BPA), a chemical used in cans and plastics, can seep into the foods and beverages inside. In lab studies, BPA affects animal hormone levels (but weren't shown to be harmful). In 2010, the FDA announced plans to study how BPA affects infants, who are exposed to higher levels of BPA from plastic baby bottles and feeding cups. In 2008, an FDA panel concluded that *parabens*, chemicals that have weak estrogen activity and are used as preservatives in cosmetics and body care products, posed no risk because the amounts used are minimal and don't build up in the body.

Myths and Other Unproven Risk Factors

Despite Internet rumors, radio, television, cellular phones, microwave ovens, and power lines haven't been shown to affect cancer risk. Having an abortion or using antiperspirants, lipsticks with lead, or underwire bras don't increase breast cancer risk. You're no more likely to develop breast cancer if you use these items than women who don't use them.

THE FORCE PERSPECTIVE: LIFESTYLE DOES INFLUENCE GENETIC PREDISPOSITION

FORCE members often ask if modifying lifestyle factors can influence their high predisposition for cancer. The short answer is yes! A mutation or other factor that puts you at high risk doesn't guarantee you'll develop breast or ovarian cancer. You may not be the master of your own fate if you have a BRCA mutation, but you can certainly sway it in your favor. It's in your own best interests to do everything you can to avoid substances or behaviors that cause genetic damage, and maximize your body's ability to repair damage that does occur (by eating foods that are high in antioxidants, for example). You'll reap the added benefit of improving your mental and physical health as you age and your risk increases.

WHAT TO REMEMBER ABOUT LIFESTYLE CHOICES

- Eat a varied and primarily plant-based diet.
- If you consume dairy, choose nonfat products.
- Maintain a healthy weight to reduce risk. Exercise for at least thirty to sixty minutes most days.
- Avoid large doses of vitamin and mineral supplements unless recommended by your healthcare provider.

LEARN MORE ABOUT LIFESTYLE CHOICES

The National Center for Complementary and Alternative Medicine (http://nccam.nih.gov/health/whatiscam/) is a government information resource about the safety and effectiveness of complementary and alternative medicines, based on scientific study.

The New American Plate emphasizes satisfying foods that promote health, balance weight, and reduce the risk for disease (www.aicr.og, click on "The New American Plate").

Mindless Eating: Why We Eat More than We Think, by Brian Wansink, Ph.D. (http://www.mindlesseating.org), explains how to control emotional factors that prompt us to eat when we're not hungry.

The Centers for Disease Control also provide information about weight loss and fitness (www.cdc.gov/physicalactivity/everyone/guidelines).

Chapter 15   Sharing Information

with Friends, Family,

and Coworkers

ALTHOUGH ISSUES RELATED to hereditary predisposition are deeply personal, the decisions you make may affect others. Sharing with loved ones along the way can help you shoulder the burden of hereditary risk and gain new perspective about testing, risk management, diagnosis, and treatment. It may not be easy. These are complex issues, and family dynamics can make these conversations difficult.

Sharing Risk and Genetic Testing Information with Family

Your family members may already be familiar with genetic counseling and testing. Perhaps you've already had conversations with them about cancer or risk, or a relative has accompanied you to healthcare appointments. If not, requesting information to build your family medical history is a good way to introduce the subject. If you're tested for a mutation, your results may benefit your relatives. If you test positive, share this information with your family, because they may have the same mutation and high risk. You needn't share your complete medical records and details with everyone if you prefer not to; your genetic counselor can identify information that will be most helpful to others and with which relatives you should share results. It will be helpful to disclose the type of mutation you have—a 187delAG mutation in the BRCA1 gene, for example—so if relatives decide to be tested, the lab will know what to look for. Consider not just the impact of learning that cancer runs in your family, but also the potential risk of not disclosing information.

Table 15. Information-sharing worksheet

Sharing information with your first-generation family
(mother/father/siblings/children)

Relative	What to share	How to share	When to share	Notes
_____	_____	_____	_____	____
_____	_____	_____	_____	____

There's never a good time to learn that hereditary disease runs in your family or that you might be genetically predisposed to one cancer or another. It's important, however, to share what you find with other members of your family. Not all people want to know whether they have a mutation, but the decision to ignore inherited risk or take action against it should be their own. Considering what to say and how to say it may help you have a more successful conversation. Documenting the following information will help you collect your thoughts about what you want to share with family members and how best to do it. Create separate documents for discussions with your first-generation, second-generation, and third-generation relatives. (You can download and print the form illustrated in table 15 from the FORCE website.)

Coping with Family Dynamics

The loving support of those close to you can help you deal with hereditary cancer and high risk. The challenges of the situation often forge a stronger family bond and foster improved communication. Your risk management decisions may be unconditionally supported, particularly if cancer is already a much-discussed topic. For many families, the opposite is true. Not everyone appreciates knowing that they may have an unusually high cancer risk, and because the subject is disturbing, it may generate conflict. Some people prefer the ostrich approach, keeping their heads in the sand when bad news arrives, and you may not be able to change their minds.

Ideally, these issues are best approached as a family, when dialogue is nonthreatening and concerns are voiced openly. That's not always possible, and you may feel tense or unsure about approaching the subject. The most effective way to share medical information depends on your relationship with relatives and how well they communicate with you and each other. If your family has pre-existing conflict, consider involving a professional counselor, trusted friend, or other neutral third party to help facilitate productive communication. Be straightforward. This can be difficult, especially if your relationships aren't cordial. You may need to approach family members in different ways, depending on your level of closeness or estrangement. If you don't know what to say, try something like, "I just learned some medical information that affects our family's risk for disease. May I share it with you?" or "I was tested for a hereditary mutation and I have my results—are you interested?" rather than "I have a genetic mutation—you and your kids must be tested too."

If you have a family organizer or conduit—the person who always seems to know what's going on with everyone and passes the information along to others—you may want to speak with her first. It may be more difficult if you've been out of touch. If you haven't been in contact with your cousins for twenty years, how do you call them out of the blue to say they may have a dangerously high cancer risk? When it isn't possible or desirable to speak face-to-face with distant or estranged family members, call, send a letter, or e-mail. Clarify how you're related, if necessary, and explain that you have medical information that may be relevant to their health. Provide them with the names of genetics specialists in their area so that they can get credible information and make their own informed decisions about genetic testing. Your genetic counselor can provide letters and information packets as examples of what to include.

It's difficult to share your test results and risk management decisions with people who argue, aren't interested, or tell you what you're planning is wrong. Some people may respond with anger, suspicion, or a barrage of questions you're unprepared to answer. Conflict may also arise when the information is perceived as upsetting or useless. The realization of your risk may scare them. One parent may agree with your course of action while the other considers it too drastic or feels guilty and avoids the topic altogether. A sister who has struggled through breast cancer treatment may tell you to proceed full steam ahead with surgery. Another who hasn't may consider it too drastic. Well-intentioned loved ones might try to protect you by dismissing your fears or telling you to think positively. They may be afraid for you or not want to see you unhappy. It's natural for the people who care about you to reassure you; it may be equally important for you to have a confidante with whom you can share and vent your fears. The input of others is helpful to gain perspective, but ultimately, risk management decisions are yours and yours alone.

Realize that others may not know as much as you do about hereditary cancer. They may be confused or put off by terms they don't understand. Give relatives a chance to absorb what you've told them. If they feel forced to give opinions before they've absorbed shocking news, they may respond differently than if they have a chance to think about it and understand how they feel. If others in your family subsequently test positive, avoid pressuring them to make the same decision you did, and respect their right to gather information and make their own informed decisions. Be supportive without being insistent.

MY STORY: Sharing Information with Patience and Gentle Encouragement

After I tested positive for a BRCA1 mutation, I felt a responsibility to share my information with my uncle and cousins. I gave my uncle our family's medical history, suggested he might want to be tested, and gave him information about genetic counselors in his area. He asked that I not share the information with my cousins before he had time to review it. As time passed, I began online contact with a cousin, although I never asked if he knew anything about our family's mutation, because I wanted to respect my uncle's request. I felt my cousins needed to make their own informed decisions. I wasn't sure what I should do. I followed up with my uncle and carefully emphasized how his own genetic counseling would give my cousins information they deserved to have. He did see a genetic counselor and was tested—he doesn't have the mutation. I was ready to tell him that I would speak to my cousins about this against his wishes if he didn't share the information. Happily, that wasn't necessary. —CATHY

Asking a Relative to Be Tested

When a mutation hasn't been identified in a family, genetic counselors identify who should be tested first to maximize information for all family members. This might not be you, even if you were the only one in the family to have genetic counseling. Asking someone else in the family to test first can be particularly challenging if you're not close to them or if they're uninterested. They might be concerned about health, privacy, insurance, or other issues, or upset or confused about genetic information they've received from people who aren't trained in genetics. Relatives are more likely to pursue testing when they understand how their results can benefit them and others in the family. The best way to ensure they receive balanced and credible information is to direct them to a genetics expert.

When a Relative Asks You to Be Tested

If you've had ovarian, fallopian tube, primary peritoneal, pancreatic, or breast cancer (especially if diagnosed before age 50), you may be the most appropriate person in the family to initiate genetic testing. It's a decision that is best made with credible and up-to-date information provided by a genetics expert.

MY STORY: I Don't Want to Talk about It

When I learned I carried a BRCA mutation, the last thing I wanted to do was talk about it. The thought of telling my closest friends made my stomach turn. So I hid the piece of paper that said "positive for a deleterious

(continued)

mutation" and did everything possible to forget that I was basically a tick-ing time bomb. They give you the information and then they say, "Don't panic. Don't be neurotic. Don't be paranoid." But your body can go off at anytime, and that pressure starts right away.   —JOANNA

Issues for Spouses, Partners, and People You Date

Telling your partner or spouse about your high risk or your plans to deal with it can strongly affect a relationship. While devastating news can unravel a relationship with weak foundations, it often strengthens the caring bond two people share. In a study of young single women who had genetic testing before marriage, participants reported fear and anxiety prior to sharing their BRCA mutation status with dating partners. Yet many of the women felt that sharing their status had positive effects on their relationships.[1]

A partner who seems uninterested or uncaring may be fearful, particularly if this is the first experience with a serious health issue. He may be afraid of losing you. Often partners feel distressed by a medical issue because they have no control over it and can't fix it. They don't know how to deal with something that disrupts their normal lives, so they ignore it. Your tone and attitude make a difference. Calmly explain the circumstances. Talk honestly about what you need and how he can best support you. Talk about how your oophorectomy may affect your plans for children, what breast reconstruction involves, or what side effects you might expect from chemoprevention. Invite your partner to participate in your research, doctor visits, and decisions. Although it's your body, the life disruptions caused by a BRCA mutation affect you both, and hopefully, you'll overcome these issues together.

Sexuality, Intimacy, and Body Image

For most of us, sexuality and sensuality are intertwined, bound together by the intimacy we feel with another person. When life throws us a curve (like inheriting a BRCA mutation) and disrupts our normal lives, shared intimacy is often one of the first casualties. Preventive choices or the aftermath of radiation, chemotherapy, chemoprevention, or surgery may shake your otherwise confident feelings about your body image, self esteem, libido, and ultimately your ability to be sexually satisfied. Intimacy may be the last thing on your mind as you cope with mammograms, MRIs, biopsies, or hot flashes after your oophorectomy. If you've had a mastectomy, you may dread that first moment of naked intimacy: the revelation that your breasts are gone or that your reconstructed breasts can't sense your partner's touch.

If you're dating, do you drop the genetic bomb early in the relationship ("Hi. My name is Kim. I don't have breasts.") or wait until you feel comfortable with each other? Trust your instincts to know when the time is right. Discuss your loss of libido before it becomes a stumbling block between the two of you. Talk openly with your partner, who probably shares your anxiety but may not volunteer opinions or feelings until prompted. At first, your partner may be afraid to touch your reconstructed breasts. If you have reduced breast sensation, find other methods of stimulation and pleasure. If you feel emotionally removed from your physical self, reconnect by learning the positives of your new body. Relax to ease your anxieties. Don't be afraid to look for new ways to achieve what you want.

Keeping your emotional and physical bonds strong may depend more on your actions than your partner's, who'll likely respond to your attitude toward intimacy.

SIX TIPS FOR TALKING WITH YOUR CHILDREN

1. Use simple, age-appropriate terms to explain concepts and to answer your child's questions.

2. Validate your child's concerns. Pushing a child's fears aside makes the situation appear too big and scary to talk about.

3. Realize your feelings are separate from your child's, which may be very different.

4. Avoid unrealistic promises. Broken promises can diminish trust.

5. Allow your child to tell you how little or how much she wants to know. Some children are more curious; others are more private.

6. Respect your children's own life path and their decisions about being tested.

Source: Adapted from the Parenting at a Challenging Time Program at Massachusetts General Hospital (www.mghpact.org).

Give yourself time to become comfortable with your body after surgery or treatment. Practice positive self-talk: "I'm the same woman I have always been," "I am strong and beautiful," or "I am loved." It can change how you feel about intimacy. For women who feel a loss of sexuality, the road back to sexual confidence and comfort often begins with touching, hugging, and caressing. Rather than focusing on the end result (satisfying sexual encounters), rely on love and affection to nurture your relationship. Be patient; the rest will follow. You can be satisfied—the way you achieve that satisfaction might be different. Remember that you're the same person, and you're so much more than the sum of your parts. Despite these changes, you can achieve satisfying and fulfilling intimacy after cancer, treatment, or surgery. If you need help to reclaim your healthy relationship and body image, speak with a certified sexual counselor.

EXPERT VIEW: What Should You Tell Your Children about Cancer and Risk?

BY KAREN HURLEY, PH.D.

It's natural to want to protect your kids from difficult topics, and it may feel less distressing in the short run to act like everything's fine. However, children can pick up on adult distress without understanding what's happening, and they can be sensitive to subtle changes in routine, such as hushed phone conversations, increased doctor appointments, or preoccupation with big decisions. In the long run, well-intentioned efforts to shield children can undermine their trust. Instead, provide simple, realistic information that matches your child's cognitive and coping abilities, realizing that each child might need a different approach depending on age, maturity level, temperament, or other life stressors.

It's also natural to put your child's well-being first, but make sure you tend to your own stress level as well. Communication about risk may be particularly complicated by guilty feelings about the possibility of passing on a mutation. Guilt is a common response to uncontrollable events, and you may blame yourself, even though you know intellectually that genetic inheritance is completely random. A good antidote is to take control of teaching your children about coping with life's difficulties. You can pass on a legacy of resilience, empowerment, and love that helps them deal not only with cancer risk in the family, but with any challenge that life has to offer.

What Should You Tell Employers and Coworkers?

Deciding who to tell and what to tell them depends on your relationships with individuals at work. The corporate culture in your workplace and how you feel about your coworkers will guide what you share with them. If your coworkers are like family, as many are, you may want to tell them about your surgery or why you've been preoccupied. If you're not particularly close with any of them, you needn't disclose your high-risk status or divulge information. You'll need to explain to your boss why you need time off (to recover from surgery, for example) and how long you'll be away, or why certain symptoms affect your productivity or ability to do your job. You may hesitate to share information because you don't want to be treated differently or you would rather avoid the gossip mill. Set boundaries around how much you want to share and with whom. Your demeanor and attitude when you share your situation often sets the stage for how others respond. Your coworkers may be quite supportive of your decisions. On the other hand, if you make it clear you don't want any extra attention, you probably won't get any.

DEALING WITH NAYSAYERS AND THE UNSUPPORTIVE

Gandhi said, "I will not let anyone walk through my mind with their dirty feet," and neither should you. This includes people who neither understand nor support your decisions. You're fortunate if everyone you encounter encourages your choices—that doesn't always happen. Not everyone will appreciate the risk you face or the challenge of making decisions when there are no great choices. Some people may question whether you're truly at high risk or may be of the impression that cancer can be cured, so why worry about it? No matter how close someone is to you, she can't possibly know what it's like to walk in your shoes unless she's had to make the same decisions. You may hear outrageously inappropriate comments, such as, "You must come to your senses!" or "How can I stop you from dismembering your body?" Be prepared with a positive comeback or avoid these people altogether. Don't let naysayers sway your certainty that what you're doing is right for you.

EMPLOYMENT LAWS AND PRIVACY ISSUES

The Genetic Information Nondiscrimination Act prohibits employers from discriminating on the basis of genetic information or a genetic test result. Employers may not request your genetic information or use it to make decisions involving hiring, firing, job assignments, or promotions. Some exceptions apply, including an exemption for businesses with fewer than fifteen employees.

THE FORCE PERSPECTIVE: ASKING FOR HELP

Asking for help can be difficult, especially if you're used to being healthy, strong, and self-sufficient. Women often tell us they feel disturbed by misguided reactions to their genetic circumstances:

"Why have my friends abandoned me during the hardest time of my life?"

"Why doesn't my sister (partner/spouse/friend) know what I need?"

"How can my father be so insensitive?"

Sometimes people say nothing because they're afraid to say the wrong thing. At times, people say the wrong thing because they don't want to be silent. They want to support you; they just don't know how. Facing cancer risk or cancer itself is not the time to be stoic. It's a loving kindness to ask people for help and to let them know exactly what you need.

WHAT TO REMEMBER ABOUT SHARING INFORMATION

- Share your medical information, including genetic test results, with family members, especially if you're positive. They may have the same mutation and high risk for cancer.
- Don't assume your relatives are already informed about genetic predisposition or that they might not want to know.
- Even those close to you may strongly disagree with your risk management strategies.
- Explain genetic risk and preventive actions in age-appropriate terms to your children.

LEARN MORE ABOUT SHARING INFORMATION

Find a certified sexual counselor at the American Association of Sexuality Educators, Counselors, and Therapists (www.aasect.org).

Sexuality and Fertility after Cancer, by Leslie R. Schover, is a comprehensive resource for survivors.

A Tiny Boat at Sea, by Izetta Smith (www.compassionbooks.com), and *In Mommy's Garden*, by Neyal Ammary (available at no charge at www.cancercare.org), explain how to help children whose parent has cancer. The helpful ideas also apply to previvor parents.

Chapter 16 Young and at High Risk

ANYONE DEALING WITH HEREDITARY CANCER ISSUES has special concerns and challenges, no matter what her age. If you're a young woman, you face additional uncertainties surrounding the risk and reality of cancer at a time in your life when you have fewer resources and probably have little experience with serious disease. You may be working hard to position yourself professionally or start a family or you may already have young children. Although most women diagnosed with breast or ovarian cancer are 50 or older, your genetic predisposition translates to high risk before that age and increased risk even during your twenties and thirties.

Should You Consider Testing Now?
Young Previvors

If cancer runs in your family, will you benefit from being tested now? If you test positive, you'll face complex decisions. How do you balance the concern of developing cancer with a lifetime of high-risk surveillance, chemoprevention with life-changing side effects, or body-altering surgery? You may struggle to determine whether you should have prophylactic mastectomies to reduce your risk, and question the best time to do so. Your healthcare team can help you sort through these issues, even if you're not ready to be tested now.

MY STORY: A New Understanding

If I had a crystal ball, I'm not sure I'd want to know now what the future might reveal. When I'm 18, I'll decide whether or not to be tested. No matter what my result, I'll always be a part of a family with hereditary cancer. My mom, grandmother, aunt, great-aunt, and two cousins have a BRCA mutation and have had breast cancer. Cancer is the furthest thing from the minds of most people my age, but not for me. My family's genetic background has given me a new understanding that sets me apart from my peers. Even though it was frightening to watch my mother go through treatment, her courage comforted me. Now I see that ignoring my fears doesn't take away my risk, and none of us is invincible. Mom used to say that living with cancer risk was like having a dark cloud over her. My cloud might appear in that crystal ball. I'm pretty sure that someday, I'll have the strength to take a look. —ARIELLE

Young Women in Treatment

If you've had breast cancer and you're not yet 40, you're not alone. Although you may be the youngest person in your oncologist's office, over 250,000 young women with breast cancer have been there before you.[1] If you have breast cancer before age 50 or ovarian cancer at any age, NCCN guidelines recommend you consult with a genetic counselor and consider BRCA testing. While young previvors usually have plenty of time to consider risk management options, if you develop cancer, you need to make more immediate treatment decisions, which may be influenced by knowledge of your mutation status. Some women prefer to delay testing until they complete treatment, rather than trying to grapple with new information and decisions under pressure.

Diagnostic Difficulties

Screening high-risk women for breast cancer before age 40 with clinical breast exam, mammogram, and MRI is very effective, but it's not foolproof. Mammography is good at finding microcalcifications (changes in breast tissue that could indicate cancer); it's not as good at finding masses in the dense breast tissue seen in young women. Additionally, some experts propose that the accompanying increased lifetime exposure to radiation from starting annual mammograms before age 30 could lead to a slightly increased breast cancer risk. MRI is more sensitive to breast changes. It often finds suspicious areas that prove to be benign, increasing the chance of unnecessary biopsies.

Despite these concerns, expert guidelines recommend a combination of annual MRI and mammogram beginning at age 25 or ten years younger than the earliest breast cancer diagnosis to maximize the chances of finding breast cancer early in high-risk women. Because younger women who develop breast cancer often discover it themselves when they find a lump or change through breast awareness or self-exam, being aware of your body and learning proper BSE technique is equally important.[2] Don't ignore a lump, discharge, or other suspicious symptom, even if it appears in your twenties or thirties and you believe you're too young to develop breast cancer. Tell your doctor right away. Sometimes, doctors assume a young woman's symptoms are due to harmless cysts and decide to wait and see what develops. If you have a BRCA mutation or a family history of cancer, choose doctors with expertise in managing high-risk women, and make them aware of your genetic status. Have any lump or breast change thoroughly examined and preferably biopsied. Appropriate risk management is important. Talk to your healthcare team about the NCCN guidelines as described in chapter 8.

Dealing with a Diagnosis before Menopause

Treatment options are often the same regardless of your age at diagnosis. Before menopause, however, standard procedures, including surgery, radiation, chemotherapy, and hormone therapy can have a greater impact on your sexuality, self-image, and fertility.

Your treatment may cause early menopause or menopausal symptoms. You're more likely to have hot flashes and other symptoms the closer you are to natural menopause, and especially if you're in your late thirties or forties. Menopause caused by chemotherapy may be temporary or irreversible, depending on the specific medication used. Some oncologists treat premenopausal women with monthly injections of leuprolide acetate (Lupron) or goserelin (Zoladex), medications that stop your ovaries from producing estrogen. You'll go into premature menopause as a result. If you're at high risk for ovarian cancer due to a BRCA mutation or other factors, and have no plans for future pregnancies, oophorectomy is often recommended instead to permanently stop estrogen production and dramatically lower your risk for ovarian cancer.

Research shows that BRCA mutation carriers with ovarian cancer respond better to treatment and survive longer than women who don't have a mutation.[3] Your treatment will involve bilateral salpingo-oophorectomy, which will also lower your risk for breast cancer. That's important, because after treatment, you'll still have high risk for cancer in eithcr breast. You'll need routine screening according to recommended guidelines for high-risk individuals. Some ovarian cancer survivors consider having prophylactic mastectomy to lower their risk. The decision is individual and often depends on the extent of your cancer and your prognosis.

Young Menopause

If your treatment results in menopausal symptoms that just won't quit, your options for hormonal therapy are limited. Coping with hot flashes, reduced libido, and other menopausal symptoms can make young women feel they're sacrificing their youth and fertility to treat their cancer. Most oncologists won't prescribe hormones after breast or ovarian cancer. Some doctors first recommend vaginal estrogen to alleviate vaginal dry-

DEALING WITH THE EMOTIONS OF CANCER

Cancer is a challenge for anyone. It may be particularly difficult for young women, who struggle with issues their older counterparts don't face. The physical and emotional upheaval of diagnosis and treatment can be especially disorienting and disruptive. After diagnosis, you may feel anxious about your personal relationships and insecure about your body and self-image. How do you tell someone you're dating that you're losing your hair or missing a breast? What happens when you and your partner want children and that's no longer possible after treatment? If you're diagnosed before age 40, you're less likely to have peers who can relate to your experience, so it's particularly important to find resources to help you deal with these issues. Ask whether your local cancer facility has a young women's support group, visit FORCE's website, and consider the resources listed at the end of this chapter.

ness. In situations where no other remedy restores your quality of life, some oncologists may prescribe low-dose hormones if your tumor was hormone receptor–negative, you had bilateral mastectomies, and your treatment is at least three years behind you. If you're a survivor with menopausal symptoms that disrupt your life, speak with your oncologist about the benefits and risks of each option described in chapter 13.

Planning Your Family, Preserving Your Fertility

Having a BRCA mutation raises unique family planning and fertility issues that may otherwise never have surfaced. Topics you may not have thought much about, such as breastfeeding, timing of pregnancies, or choice of birth control, may take on new significance.

Birth Control

Taking oral contraceptives slightly elevates breast cancer risk in the general population. When you stop using the Pill, the increase in risk diminishes over time, reverting to average after ten years.[4] The most comprehensive study of oral contraceptives in women with BRCA mutations found increased breast cancer only among women who began taking the Pill before 1975 or before age 30, or in women who continued on contraceptives for five years or more. BRCA mutation carriers who took contraceptives for three years after age 30 had a substantially lower risk for ovarian cancer.[5] There is little long-term research on newer oral contraceptives, many of which may be less likely to raise breast cancer risk because they contain lower doses of hormones. Solid evidence shows that oral contraceptives reduce ovarian cancer risk. Tubal ligation, which is usually reversible, also prevents pregnancy. It may also lower ovarian cancer risk, yet not as much as oral contraceptives.

Fertility

Cancer treatments and preventive actions that interrupt or end fertility can be a tough pill to swallow if you look forward to future pregnancies. American Society of Clinical Oncology guidelines suggest that oncologists discuss fertility preservation and refer all patients of childbearing age to specialists.[6] If fertility is a concern, discuss your treatment options with your oncologist and ask for a referral to a fertility specialist before beginning any chemotherapy.

Several studies indicate that infertile women may be more likely to develop breast cancer, although no evidence conclusively shows that fertility medications are the cause. Clomiphene citrate (Clomid), a common fertility drug used to treat women who don't produce enough eggs to become pregnant, isn't known to increase breast or ovarian cancer risk. It has been linked to an increased chance of uterine cancer.

In Vitro Fertilization

If you're facing oophorectomy or chemotherapy and want to preserve the option to have your own biological children, you might want to explore in vitro fertilization. Your eggs can be harvested before treatment or surgery and then fertilized with your partner's sperm outside the womb (in a laboratory). The resulting embryos can be stored until you're ready to have your baby. If you still have your uterus, you can carry the embryo to term. As an alternative, if you've had a hysterectomy, a surrogate can carry the pregnancy for you.

Preimplantation Genetic Diagnosis

The *preimplantation genetic diagnosis* (PGD) procedure screens embryos to determine whether they've inherited their parents' disease or disease-causing mutation. PGD begins with in vitro fertilization. When an embryo reaches adequate size, one cell is removed and tested; this option is available to test for a BRCA mutation. Only unaffected embryos are implanted into the mother or surrogate.

Breast Cancer and Pregnancy

Breast cancer is difficult to detect during pregnancy or breastfeeding.

IS PREGNANCY SAFE AFTER BREAST CANCER?

Traditionally, doctors recommended waiting at least two years after breast cancer treatment to become pregnant, because the risk of recurrence is higher during this period. European analysis of fourteen previous trials, however, found that pregnancy may be safe for breast cancer survivors. Even though the information didn't specifically address survivors of BRCA-related breast cancers, and it hasn't been validated by long-term studies, it's encouraging for women who want to have children when their breast cancer is behind them.

Source: ECCO—the European CanCer Organisation, "Pregnancy for Breast Cancer Survivors: Meta-Analysis Reveals It Is Safe and Could Improve Survival," presented at the European Breast Cancer Conference, Barcelona, Spain, 2010.

Normal lumps and thickening can hide more serious changes, and radiation from mammograms may harm the fetus. With their high risk in mind, some previvors have prophylactic mastectomy before they become pregnant. This is a hard choice that eliminates the possibility of breastfeeding, but it provides peace of mind to focus on pregnancy without worrying about surveillance or a diagnosis.

Pregnancy-related breast cancers are often more advanced, yet moms-to-be appear to fare as well as other women during treatment, experiencing similar rates of recurrence and survival. Treatment depends on the type and stage of cancer. During the first trimester, treatment is limited to a wide excision with a local anesthetic to remove the lump; any other treatment may harm the fetus. Mastectomy performed under a general anesthetic and chemotherapy are safe by the second trimester. Radiation and hormone therapy, if needed, must wait until after the baby's birth.

Parity (Number of Births)

Studying the effects of pregnancy on BRCA-associated breast and ovarian cancer risk is difficult, because such a small percentage of the population has mutations. Initial research shows that cancer risk may depend on the type of mutation and the number of children you have. Studies have been observational, and experts can't be certain whether parity or some other factor is responsible for observed changes in risk.

Although decisions about having children are personal, cancer experts encourage BRCA carriers to complete childbearing by age 40, when the risk of ovarian cancer increases, and to remove their ovaries before cancer develops.

Breastfeeding

Breastfeeding slightly reduces the risk for sporadic breast cancer: the longer you breastfeed, the lower your risk. It may have a similar protective effect for women with BRCA1 mutations.[7] Whether it affects women with BRCA2 mutations in the same way is unclear. Although breastfeeding benefits both mother and baby, having milk in the ducts makes imaging difficult; there's no reliable way of screening until you've stopped. If you're at high risk for breast cancer, complete recommended semiannual breast surveillance before you become pregnant, if possible.

MY STORY: The Hardest Decision

I was engaged when I tested positive for BRCA1. At 31, I was approaching the age when my risk increased. Oophorectomy was recommended when I was done having children; I was unsure what to do about my breasts. I finally made up my mind; it was the hardest decision I've ever made. After my wedding, I had both breasts removed. I wanted to become pregnant, but I was concerned about screening, particularly at a time when increased estrogen could spike my risk, and an early cancer (which could be very aggressive) would be difficult to find. It was a risk I wasn't willing to take. I don't regret my decision. I was sad when I couldn't breastfeed—I was aware that breastfeeding is best for newborns and creates a strong mother-child bond. Feeding times were still special, and bonding was solid. Now that my children are almost 4 and 2, and I look at their joy and inquisitiveness, I know they are healthy. I feel confident that I'm doing everything within my power to make sure that I will be here for them for a long time. —KENDRA

Adoption after Cancer

Whether you're a cancer survivor or previvor, if you want to have children and you can't become pregnant, adoption is a wonderful way to create or expand your family. Your genetic predisposition or cancer history shouldn't preclude your approval as an adoptive parent; your doctor will need to provide an accurate assessment of your health and prognosis.

Oophorectomy in Young Women

Salpingo-oophorectomy lowers risk for ovarian and fallopian tube cancer and reduces breast cancer risk by about 50 percent. Deciding whether it's right for you—and when to have it—can be challenging. For women with mutations, most ovarian cancer risk occurs after age 50, although some women are diagnosed in their thirties or forties. Having surgery closer to age 35 increases your chances of avoiding ovarian cancer but leads to early menopause. Although waiting allows you more years with your natural hormones, it increases your risk for a diagnosis in the interim and may not give you the same reduction in breast cancer risk. Whether and when to have an oophorectomy is an individual decision that is influenced by your priorities, your tolerance for risk, and how the risks and benefits of oophorectomy apply to your circumstances.

Some women delay surgery because they're concerned about highly publicized studies that suggest women of *average risk* who remove their ovaries before menopause—particularly those who don't then take estrogen—have increased risk for heart disease, lung cancer, and early death. Other studies show that taking some types of hormones increases the risk for breast cancer. These studies, however, apply to women in the general population. Research specific to women with BRCA mutations confirms the benefits of oophorectomy. According to PROSE study data, women with mutations have a lower chance of early death after oophorectomy than women with mutations who don't have oophorectomy, and short-term hormone replacement in young previvors doesn't erase the beneficial breast cancer risk reduction of oophorectomy.[8]

Sorting through Emotions

Forced to make life choices because you're high risk, you may feel a sense of pressure to change or accelerate your life plans. How do you deal with this sense of compressed time when you're an unmarried 27-year-old who is dating? How do you discuss this with your partner or explain it to your friends—will any of them really "get" it? You may tend to face life with a seriousness uncommon in your peers. If you're feeling isolated, seek support through the FORCE website or your local FORCE group, where others who have faced these same issues can help. Intrusive thoughts, significant anxiety, insomnia, and physical symptoms such as stomachaches may indicate that you need more help or support.

EXPERT VIEW: A Young Woman's Toolkit for Emotional Health

BY KAREN HURLEY, PH.D.

- Support: Make sure you have at least one confidante who will listen attentively without judgment or an agenda of her or his own.
- Coping statements: Create a series of meaningful positive statements to coach yourself through difficult moments.
- Letting go: Distinguish between what you can and cannot control. You can change your thoughts. You can't change other people's reactions.
- Balance: Prioritize enjoyable activities that will refresh you enough to take on the next round of appointments, decisions, and responsibilities.
- Physical activity: Stay healthy and energized with exercise. It is a natural mood enhancer.
- Information thermostat: Figure out the next one thing you need to know, and then pause there before you get overwhelmed.
- Take a breath: Remember that even when the pressure is on, there is always time to take a breath. A deep breath can reconnect you with the calm, centered place from which you can make your best decisions.

INSURANCE AND PAYMENT ISSUES

If you're 40 and uninsured, check with your local hospital, YWCA, and community health organizations to see if they offer breast cancer education and screening for high-risk young women. Most insurance policies don't cover in vitro fertilization or PGD.

Some high-risk young women research their disability, life, and long-term care insurance options before they undergo genetic testing.

THE FORCE PERSPECTIVE: WHAT WOMEN THINK ABOUT PGD

For more than a decade, PGD has been used to screen embryos for cystic fibrosis, Huntington's, and other hereditary diseases, including cancer. A FORCE survey of our members showed that:

- 79 percent were unaware of PGD.
- 53 percent felt PGD was an acceptable option to combat hereditary disease.
- 33 percent would consider using PGD themselves.
- 29 percent feared PGD could be used for the wrong reasons, such as creating "designer babies."
- 2 percent were offended, feeling they wouldn't be alive if their parents had used PGD.

WHAT TO REMEMBER IF YOU'RE YOUNG AND AT HIGH RISK

- High-risk women more often develop breast cancer before age 40 than women in the general population.
- Young women face unique risk-reducing and treatment issues.
- Doctors don't always ask about the fertility concerns of young women undergoing treatment.
- It's especially important to be your own advocate when facing breast and ovarian cancer before age 40.

LEARN MORE ABOUT BEING YOUNG AND AT HIGH RISK

Livestrong Young Adult Alliance (www.livestrong.org) is a coalition of organizations dedicated to improving survival rates and quality of life for young adults with cancer.

Livestrong's Fertile Hope Initiative (www.fertilehope.org) provides reproductive information, support, and hope to cancer patients and survivors whose medical treatments may affect fertility.

Young Survival Coalition (www.youngsurvival.org) offers information and support for young women with breast cancer.

Bright Pink (www.brightpink.org) offers networking and support for young women concerned about breast cancer.

Chapter 17 How BRCA Affects Men

LIKE WOMEN, MEN CAN INHERIT BRCA MUTATIONS from either parent. And when they do, like women, they face an increased lifetime risk of certain cancers (see table 16). When men have BRCA mutations, however, their risk for breast cancer is lower than women who have the same mutation. Men should consult with a genetic counselor when they:

- have an inherited BRCA mutation in the family.
- have been diagnosed with breast cancer, young-onset prostate cancer, or pancreatic cancer.
- have prostate cancer and a family history of breast cancer or ovarian cancer.
- have male relatives who have had breast cancer.
- have female relatives who have had breast cancer, particularly before age 50, or ovarian cancer at any age.
- are of Jewish ancestry and their family history includes breast, ovarian, pancreatic, or prostate cancer.

Table 16. BRCA mutations increase a man's risk for cancer

Cancer*	BRCA1	BRCA2
Breast	✓	✓
Prostate	✓	✓
Pancreas	✓	✓
Melanoma		✓

*Degree of risk is not the same for all cancers

EXPERT VIEW: Men React Differently to Genetic Risk

BY MARY B. DALY, M.D., PH.D.

Male members of breast or ovarian cancer families are less likely to be included in family conversations about cancer risk and are less likely to be informed of test results received by their female relatives. Reasons for selective sharing of test results with predominantly female relatives include a closer bond with women than with men in the family, the desire to protect other female relatives from breast and ovarian cancer, and the hope of receiving emotional support from them. Men are more likely to use avoidance and denial strategies to cope with cancer risk in the family. Their socialization to value physical strength above all else and their reluctance to acknowledge vulnerability can challenge the recognition of genetic health threats and the need for preventive health behaviors. As a result, men may be unaware of the health implications of carrying a BRCA mutation, for themselves and for other family members. Men who choose not to undergo genetic testing may not only pass up the chance to take active steps to protect their own health, but also miss the opportunity to provide valuable cancer risk information to their children and other relatives.

Men Get Breast Cancer Too

We hear a lot about breast cancer in women, but few men are aware that they're also at risk (see table 17). Male breast cancer doesn't often happen, even among men with mutations. Malignancies in the small amount of breast tissue behind the male nipples account for fewer than two thousand total cases in the United States each year—that's about one man diagnosed for every one hundred women with the disease. Among men who develop breast cancer, about 8 percent have a BRCA mutation.[1] Any man diagnosed should consider risk assessment with a genetics expert.

Research specific to breast cancer in men with BRCA mutations is sparse. The following factors are known to increase the likelihood

Table 17. Estimated male lifetime breast cancer risk to age 80

Population	Risk (%)
Men with a BRCA1 mutation	2
Men with a BRCA2 mutation	8.4
Men with no BRCA mutation	0.1

Sources: Wolpert N, Warner E, Seminsky MF, et al., "Prevalence of BRCA1 and BRCA2 Mutations in Male Breast Cancer Patients in Canada," *Clinical Breast Cancer* 1, no. 1 (2000): 57–63, discussion 64–65; Evans DG, Susnerwala I, Dawson J, et al., "Risk of Breast Cancer in Male BRCA2 Carriers," *Journal of Medical Genetics* 47, no. 10 (2010): 710–11.

of breast cancer in men of average risk and may also affect men with mutations.

- growing older
- having family members of either gender who have breast cancer
- being alcoholic or obese, or having chronic liver disorders—conditions that raise estrogen levels
- having Klinefelter syndrome, a rare male genetic disorder that creates high estrogen levels. Men with Klinefelter are 20 to 50 times more likely to develop breast cancer than other men[2]
- having *gynecomastia*, a benign condition characterized by enlargement of male breast tissue, obesity, or other factors, may increase the risk for breast cancer

Screening and Treatment

Men approach their overall health much differently than women, often avoiding routine health screenings or regularly seeing physicians. Most men don't routinely check their breasts (see NCCN screening guidelines in table 18). If they do find a suspicious area, they're more likely than a woman in the same situation to ignore it. Any of the following symptoms may indicate a benign breast condition or breast cancer and should be reviewed right away by a physician. Early treatment can be lifesaving.

Table 18. NCCN breast cancer surveillance guidelines for men with BRCA mutations

---

Breast self-exam training and regular monthly practice

Semiannual clinical breast examination by a healthcare professional

Consider a baseline mammogram and annual mammogram if baseline shows gynecomastia or breast density

---

- a nipple that itches, is sore, is scaly, has a rash or discharge, or appears different
- a lump or thickening in the breast or chest (Breast abnormalities may be more noticeable in a man's small breast.)
- dimpling or puckering of the breast skin

Most breast malignancies found in men are invasive ductal carcinoma. Less frequently, invasive lobular carcinoma, inflammatory breast cancer, or DCIS develops. Men with breast cancer have greater risk for a malignancy in the opposite breast, particularly when diagnosed before age 50.

Tumors with the same pathology are generally treated alike, whether they occur in men or women, and survival rates are similar when treatment begins at the same stage. By the time men see a doctor, however, their tumors are often more advanced, with a poorer outcome. Clinical breast exam, mammography, ultrasound, and biopsy may all be used to detect and stage a malignancy. The first line of treatment is a

RECONSTRUCTION FOR MEN?

Male mastectomy typically removes breast tissue and a strip of skin surrounding and including the nipple. Men don't typically need reconstruction after mastectomy. A small flap reconstruction is possible, particularly when removal of a tumor in the chest wall leaves a concave chest. Nipple reconstruction, if desired, is also an option. Men interested in reconstruction should speak with a board-certified plastic surgeon who specializes in breast reconstruction.

A man with breast cancer may feel embarrassed, especially if he considers it to be a woman's disease and finds himself the only male in the oncology waiting room. If you're a male breast cancer patient, you're not alone. About two thousand men are diagnosed each year. An online or local breast cancer support group specific to men can address these concerns and help patients deal with diagnosis and treatment.

total or modified radical mastectomy with sentinel node biopsy or axillary lymph node dissection to determine whether the cancer has spread. Lumpectomy isn't usually an option because, compared to a woman, a man's tumor involves a larger proportion of his breast. Depending on stage and tumor characteristics, surgery may be followed by chemotherapy (it may also be used before surgery to shrink the tumor), and sometimes radiation. Tamoxifen is usually prescribed for five years if a tumor is ER+, as most male breast cancers are, with the potential for similar side effects experienced by women: headache, nausea, leg cramps, bladder control issues, and rashes. Megace, a drug that blocks the effect of the male hormone androgen, may be used instead. Some oncologists prefer aromatase inhibitors to block estrogen; although they work against female breast cancers, they haven't been well studied in men. They tend to thin the bones (a bisphosphonate may be prescribed to offset this side effect) and can cause stiff joints. If initial hormonal therapy fails, medications called *gonadotropin inhibitors* may be used to lower hormone levels. Breast cancers that overexpress HER2/neu may be treated with trastuzumab (Herceptin) and chemotherapy.

MY STORY: Thriving after BRCA and Breast Cancer

I'm an 81-year-old father of four and grandfather of six. None of these is an unusual accomplishment except that I'm also a seven-year survivor of breast cancer. I found the lump while showering. A mastectomy followed, as did a bout with bladder cancer. And prostate cancer. And skin cancer. After my breast cancer diagnosis and learning I was BRCA2 positive, my four children were tested. True to the 50/50 chance of inheriting my mutation, two were positive, two were negative. I'm still here, surviving and thriving—it's entirely possible.

Most people don't know that men can get breast cancer. My advice to other men is to get in the shower and run your hands all over yourself. And if any family members have had breast cancer, go get the BRCA test. It's a simple blood test that may save your life or the life of someone you love. —GUY

High Risk for Prostate Cancer

Prostate cancer is the most commonly diagnosed cancer in North American men—and in men with BRCA mutations—and the second leading cause of male cancer deaths. In most cases in the general population, it's a particularly slow-growing disease, and most men die with it, not because of it. That's not always the case with men who have a BRCA2 mutation—their lifetime risk is particularly high: about 1 in 3; the average man's risk is 1 in 6. BRCA2-related prostate cancer may develop before age 50, is more aggressive, and has a poorer prognosis.

Early prostate cancer usually shows no symptoms. Most doctors routinely recommended an annual *prostate-specific antigen* (PSA) blood test to screen men over age 50 until a 2009 study showed that, based on PSA results, more than 1 million men in the United States were overtreated for tumors that grew too slowly to do harm.[3] This is significant, because up to one-third suffer from incontinence, impotence, and other life-affecting side effects—not from the cancer, but from treatment. This study prompted the American Cancer Society to modify its recommendations. Current guidelines (which are complex) for the general population of men advise against PSA testing until they talk with their doctors and have enough information to make an informed decision about whether to have the test. The discussion is recommended at:

- age 50 for men of average risk who are expected to live at least ten more years.
- age 45 for African American men and those who have a first-degree relative diagnosed with prostate cancer before age 65.
- age 40 for men with several first-degree relatives who had prostate cancer before age 65.

These guidelines are inadequate for BRCA2 mutation carriers, who may be more likely to die from their prostate cancer since it has a higher likelihood of being aggressive. The NCCN recommends a PSA test and baseline digital rectal exam for all men with BRCA mutations, starting at age 40. The international IMPACT study is comparing the benefit of prostate screening in men ages 40 to 69 who have BRCA mutations with those who don't. Study results (expected in 2020) will clarify the benefits of prostate cancer screening in high-risk men. Initial study findings suggest that PSA screening is effective in BRCA mutation carriers: an elevated PSA more likely signified prostate cancer in their biopsy, they were less likely to undergo a biopsy for an unfounded reason, and their cancers were generally more aggressive, requiring treatment.[4] Enroll or follow the study online (www.impact-study.co.uk).

Otherwise healthy men who are diagnosed before age 60 with cancer confined to the prostate are usually treated with *prostatectomy* (removal of the prostate gland) or radiation (either external radiation over several weeks or via one-time *brachytherapy*, which plants radioactive seeds in the prostate). Erectile dysfunction and urinary incontinence may result from either treatment. When surgery isn't an option or when an advanced tumor is contained in the prostate, cryosurgery may be used to freeze the gland to kill the cancer. It's unclear whether this procedure works as well as surgery or radiation in the long term, and side effects depend on the surgeon's skill.

FAMILY PLANNING

Like women, men can pass their BRCA mutation to their children. Some couples choose preimplantation genetic diagnosis with in vitro fertilization to selectively identify and implant embryos that don't have the mutation.

Androgen deprivation therapy may also be used. Although it doesn't cure prostate cancer, it successfully reduces tumor size and slows its growth, sometimes for several years, by suppressing hormones made in the testicles. This option lowers the level of testosterone and other male hormones. Hormone therapy can also cause many side effects, including impotence, diminished or absent libido, reduced muscle mass, weight gain, fatigue, anemia, osteoporosis, and others. These side effects can affect quality of life, and doctors disagree about whether hormone therapy harms more than it helps. Chemotherapy may be prescribed for advanced prostate cancer that doesn't respond to hormone treatment. In preliminary research, PARP inhibitors, the same experimental drugs designed to treat BRCA-related breast and ovarian tumors, effectively treated BRCA-related prostate cancers.[5]

Older men diagnosed with early stage cancer that is confined to the prostate may prefer to forego surgery and radiation, opting instead for "watchful waiting," regular checkups to monitor the progression of their disease. If a CT or MRI scan subsequently shows enlarged lymph nodes, a fine needle aspiration or a lymph node dissection of nodes in the groin can determine whether the cancer has spread. Given the potentially more aggressive nature of BRCA2-related prostate cancer, men with this mutation should speak with an oncologist who has expertise in hereditary cancer before deciding against treatment.

Do Lifestyle Changes Make a Difference?

Researchers are trying to determine whether certain foods protect against prostate cancer. Several studies suggest that eating fatty fish may be helpful. One large investigation linked eating salmon or other fatty fish more than three times weekly with reduced risk, particularly of metastatic prostate cancer: risk decreased 24 percent for each additional half-gram of fatty acids consumed daily from food (not from supplements).[6] The effect wasn't as strong when other foods were the source of fatty acids. Studies of pomegranate extract to aid in treatment for prostate cancer are also ongoing. No studies have explored the potential benefit of these foods specifically in BRCA mutation carriers.

MY STORY: Living Optimistically with BRCA

I grew up thinking a lot about breast cancer, since my mom was diagnosed when she was 38. At 7 years old, I didn't understand what it meant: she had a mastectomy, then recovered. I thought nothing about her having only one breast. Ten years later, a pattern of early onset breast cancer emerged from her father's side of the family. Mom had a recurrence and another mastectomy, and her uncle and cousin were also diagnosed. Their family tree

(continued)

showed breast, ovarian, and stomach cancers among men and women. Mom then learned that she had a BRCA2 mutation. I was stunned when I also tested positive; I didn't know what my future held. Now I needed to consider my own risk for prostate cancer, pancreatic cancer, and breast cancer. I began living a very healthy lifestyle, eating ten fruits and vegetables a day and running 35 miles a week. I'm now training for my sixth marathon. Combined with annual physicals and prostate exams, I'm in good stead for the future, and five years after receiving my test result, I'm more optimistic about what it means to live with a BRCA2 mutation. —RICHARD

Other BRCA-Related Cancers

Like their female counterparts, men with BRCA mutations have increased risk for pancreatic cancer compared to less than 1 percent in the general population. At this time, no routine screening is available, but studies are under way. Men with mutations in BRCA2 have a slightly increased risk for melanoma of the skin and eyes. They should routinely examine themselves to discover new moles or unusual changes and consider yearly exams by a dermatologist who has expertise in diagnosing skin cancer. Annual eye exams by an ophthalmologist, including pupil dilation and thorough examination of the retina, are also recommended because some forms of melanoma affect the eyes.

INSURANCE AND PAYMENT ISSUES

Men may have more difficulty getting insurance coverage for genetic testing. Policies vary, and in some cases, testing is covered only when action steps are planned based on the results—if a man intends to use the results in conjunction with PGD or in vitro fertilization, for example. Medicare covers genetic testing for men only after they've been diagnosed with cancer. Insurance company rules about coverage may change if the IMPACT study and other research show that testing men detects cancers earlier and saves lives. If you're a high-risk man without healthcare insurance or if your policy doesn't cover regular PSA tests or genetic testing, check with your local cancer society or hospital about low-cost screenings or free testing in your area.

THE FORCE PERSPECTIVE:

MORE MEN + MORE RESEARCH = MORE ANSWERS

We need to learn much more about hereditary cancer in women, and we know even less about men who inherit mutations. Yet there is good reason to believe that better screening, prevention, and treatment options could improve longevity for men with mutations. The answers we need will result only from well-conducted studies. Because men's cancer risk is not as great as women's, less research has focused on men who have BRCA mutations. Recruiting men for this research is challenging; fewer men have genetic testing, so fewer are aware they have a mutation. A FORCE study developed in collaboration with BRCA researchers is identifying the types of cancers that develop in male mutation carriers and creating a database of men who are willing to participate in research.

WHAT TO REMEMBER ABOUT HOW BRCA AFFECTS MEN

- Having a BRCA mutation, especially in BRCA2, increases a man's risk for several cancers.
- Although rare, breast cancer does occur in men.
- BRCA-related prostate cancer may be more aggressive than sporadic prostate cancer and should be treated by an oncologist who is familiar with hereditary cancers.
- Men can inherit a BRCA mutation and pass it down to their sons or daughters just as women can.

LEARN MORE ABOUT HOW BRCA AFFECTS MEN

Visit the FORCE online men's support group (www.facingourrisk.org).

Malecare (www.malecare.com) provides information on prostate cancer, testicular cancer, and male breast cancer, as well as the sexual side effects of cancer treatment.

The John W. Nick Foundation (www.malebreastcancer.org) has information about male breast cancer.

Us Too (www.ustoo.org) provides support for men affected by prostate cancer.

Chapter 18 **Diagnosis**

Hereditary Cancer

JUST TWO GENERATIONS AGO, cancers were rarely discovered until they were well advanced, almost always with dismal outcome. There is still much we don't know, but treatment is becoming more sophisticated, more personalized, and much more successful. Discovering that all cancers aren't the same has expanded our arsenal of postdiagnosis tools. Although facing cancer is never easy, treatments are less invasive, less toxic, and more tolerable.

For most women with breast cancer, the disease is discovered early and is no longer a death sentence. In the United States, over 2.5 million breast cancer survivors attest to improved methods of prevention, detection, and treatment. Although screening for ovarian cancer remains unreliable, we're finding more early stage tumors when women have prophylactic surgery. And even though most ovarian cancers are advanced by the time symptoms develop, newer, less toxic treatments allow women to live longer with fewer side effects and better quality of life.

How Important Is a Second Opinion?

It's always wise to get a second opinion about diagnosis and treatment; most insurance plans cover the cost. Gather your medical records and find a specialist by contacting your local American Cancer Society or the NCI's Cancer Information Service (www.cancer.gov/help, or 800-4-CANCER). In almost all cases, briefly delaying treatment to get another opinion isn't a problem. Let your doctor know you'd like a second opinion and ask when your treatment must begin.

Treating Hereditary Cancers
Chemotherapy

For many women, chemotherapy is the most frightening aspect of cancer. The thought of being fatigued and nauseated, losing your hair, and having your life generally disrupted isn't pleasant. Dealing with side effects may require additional treatment—medications can curb nausea, stabilize white cell count, and help to maintain your strength. Yet chemotherapy saves lives. Newer therapies target mainly cancer cells and have fewer undesirable effects, leaving healthy cells to perform their normal functions. *Neoadjuvant* (before surgery) chemotherapy is often used to shrink a large tumor so that surgery doesn't need to be as extensive. *Adjuvant* (after surgery) treatment targets remaining cancer cells.

Two tests improve the traditional trial-and-error approach to breast cancer chemotherapy, helping doctors determine which early stage cancers will most likely recur and will therefore benefit from chemo treatments—an example of how treatment is becoming more personalized. Using a sample of tumor tissue from your lumpectomy or mastectomy, OncoType DX examines twenty-one different genes and is recommended for stage 1 ER/PR+ invasive breast cancers. The MammaPrint test works similarly for tumors smaller than five centimeters—that's half of all breast cancer diagnoses—and assesses seventy genes that influence tumor progression in ER/PR+ and ER/PR– tumors. (These prognostic tests look only at gene changes that have occurred in the tumor. They aren't the same as testing for inherited BRCA mutations that are present in all the body's cells.) If you have invasive breast cancer, ask your oncologist during your preliminary consultation if you meet guidelines for either test before you decide on a course of treatment. Some health insurers may pay for a portion or all of either test. If you're uninsured or can't afford the full cost, contact the test manufacturers (www.agendia.com and www.oncotypedx.com) about their financial assistance programs.

Platinum drugs are chemotherapies frequently used for ovarian cancer and less often for breast cancer. They weaken or destroy malignant cells by interfering with their ability to repair DNA damage. Cisplatin and carboplatin are particularly effective against ovarian cancers. Although they're not generally used as first-line treatment in breast cancer, some research suggests that platinum drugs may be particularly effective against cancers in people with BRCA mutations. In a small trial, nine of ten women with BRCA1 mutations who were treated with neoadjuvant cisplatin for stage 1 to stage 3 breast cancers had a pathologically complete response—their tumors shrank until they were no longer visible.[1]

PARP Inhibitors

A new class of targeted drugs called PARP inhibitors holds promise for BRCA-related cancers. These medications block poly (ADP-ribose) polymerase proteins, substances used by cells to repair DNA damage. They appear to be especially effective at preventing cancer cells from repairing themselves once they're damaged by chemotherapy, with less effect on healthy cells—a great advantage over traditional chemotherapy, which indiscriminately targets all rapidly growing cells. This selective targeting means fewer side effects and quicker recovery.

PARPis performed well in three clinical trials. They benefited women with metastasized triple-negative breast cancer, a common type of breast cancer among African American women and women with BRCA1 mutations. Individuals who took PARPis intravenously along with chemo had improved responses—the drugs slowed progression of their cancers and the women lived longer—compared to those who received chemotherapy alone.[2] Two of the studies involved women with BRCA mutations whose metastatic breast cancer or recurrent ovarian cancer had progressed after previous chemotherapy. Both groups benefited from PARP inhibitors taken orally without chemotherapy, compared to women who had chemotherapy alone.[3] The drugs were effective and well tolerated whether participants had mutations in BRCA1 or in BRCA2, and most side effects were mild. Not all participants with BRCA mutations and advanced cancer responded this way.

Early research of PARPis for prostate and pancreatic cancer is also promising. These studies are exciting, but more large-scale research is needed to determine whether PARP inhibitors prevent return of early stage cancers and slow progression of advanced cancers. If successful, these medications might become an entirely new way of treating inherited cancers and will likely be combined with chemotherapy treatment. Even with favorable trials, it could take years before they're available outside clinical trials.

EXPERT VIEW: The Power of PARP Inhibitors

BY ANDREW TUTT, MB.CHB., PH.D., M.R.C.P., F.R.C.R.

When the location and then sequence of the BRCA1 and BRCA2 breast and ovarian cancer predisposition genes became known in the mid 1990s, much work followed to understand the function of these genes and why they lead to such high and early cancer risks. In Professor Alan Ashworth's laboratory in the U.K., we found that these genes help a type of DNA repair called homologous recombination. We began to test a theory suggested by experiments: that DNA damage from particular chemotherapies might work effectively against BRCA-related cancers. Our group and the laboratory of Dr. Tomas Helleday (another U.K. research group) explored using a drug that stopped other forms of DNA repair in cancer cells but did not affect normal cells. Only when this drug effect was combined with the BRCA1 or BRCA2 repair defect in cancer cells would there be a lethal combination that might kill the malignant cells while having little effect on normal cells. Generally, this proved to be true for PARP inhibitors. Since then, we have worked with colleagues in clinical trials using PARP inhibitors with very promising results. Several PARP inhibitor agents from different pharmaceutical companies are being tested to treat advanced BRCA1- and BRCA2-associated cancers.

Making Breast Cancer Treatment Decisions

Anyone treated for cancer hopes they'll never again face that experience, yet it can happen. Another diagnosis can be even more disrupting and disheartening than the first time around. Your treatment, even the type of chemotherapy used, may be different, depending on the nuances of your cancer: its stage, how you were treated before, and other variables.

By now you know that your high-risk status increases your risk of future cancers and may affect your treatment decisions (see table 19).

Table 19. Treatment decisions for women at high risk

Lumpectomy and radiation or mastectomy	If you're at high risk and are newly diagnosed with breast cancer, you have elevated risk for another primary cancer in either breast, even after lumpectomy and radiation. In this situation, knowing your BRCA status right away can help you decide between lumpectomy and radiation or mastectomy. (Genetic testing can be expedited for an additional fee.) Survival rates are the same with either procedure; mutation carriers who choose mastectomy are less likely to develop a second breast cancer.
Unilateral or bilateral mastectomy	Compared to women with sporadic breast cancer, women with BRCA1 mutations develop contralateral breast cancer almost five times more often, and BRCA2 mutation carriers three times more often. If you have a BRCA mutation, your surgeon or oncologist may recommend a breast MRI to determine whether you have tumors in your opposite breast. If you do, bilateral mastectomy may be the preferred treatment.
Oophorectomy or menopause-inducing medication	If you're a premenopausal BRCA mutation carrier with advanced hormone receptor–positive breast cancer and your treatment recommendation includes menopause-inducing drugs and AIs, you may want to consider combining the medications with oophorectomy instead. A small observational study showed that BRCA1 mutation carriers who had oophorectomy within six months of their breast cancer diagnosis had a higher survival rate compared to those who retained their ovaries.

Source: Møller P, Borg A, Evans DG, et al., "Survival in Prospectively Ascertained Familial Breast Cancer: Analysis of a Series Stratified by Tumour Characteristics, BRCA Mutations and Oophorectomy," *International Journal of Cancer* 101, no. 6 (2002): 555–59.

Ovarian Cancer Issues

If you're diagnosed with ovarian cancer, your treatment may include more than one type of therapy, depending on your response. Unlike some early stage breast cancers, epithelial ovarian cancers, even those found at stage 1, are usually treated with chemotherapy, and progress is often monitored with CA-125 tests.

Survival

Women with BRCA mutations who develop ovarian cancer tend to fare better than their counterparts with sporadic ovarian tumors: in some studies, they had higher five-year survival rates. Researchers aren't certain whether this is due to different tumor traits or simply a better response to chemotherapy. Survival rates among women diagnosed at stages 1 or 2 were not significantly different; BRCA mutation carriers diagnosed at stage 3 or 4 were 28 percent less likely to die compared to women who had similar stage sporadic cancer. Having either mutation increased median survival by sixteen months.[4] Other studies echo this conclusion.

Breast Cancer Risk after Ovarian Cancer

If you're a survivor of BRCA-related ovarian cancer, you have greater risk for breast cancer than other ovarian cancer survivors who don't have a mutation. It's very important to recognize and manage this high risk after your recovery. Gynecologic oncologists often recommend breast surveillance initially for their ovarian cancer patients. Some ovarian cancer survivors choose prophylactic bilateral mastectomy.

MY STORY: Survival Is What Matters

To say cancer doesn't matter is a lie. It sucks. But in spite of how awful it is to feel less than female, being alive is what matters. It may not be the ideal life you want, but it's life. You don't mess with that.   —LINDA

Ovarian Cancer Risk after Breast Cancer

If you're a breast cancer survivor with a BRCA mutation, you're at high risk for ovarian cancer. One study found the ten-year risk after breast cancer to be 13 percent for BRCA1 mutation carriers and 7 percent for women with a mutation in BRCA2.[5] Another study found that a quarter of the deaths in BRCA mutation carriers who had early stage breast cancer was due to subsequent ovarian cancer.[6] Your risk is also elevated (it's unclear how much) if you have a family history of breast and ovarian cancer, even if you don't have a BRCA mutation. If your family has multiple members with breast cancer, but no history of ovarian cancer and no known BRCA mutation, your lifetime risk for ovarian cancer is estimated to be the same as an average woman's (1.4 percent).[7]

MY STORY: My Preventive Surgery Found Cancer

My sister, a nurse practitioner, knew instantly that the mass on my father's chest was breast cancer. Treatment and genetic testing followed, confirming a BRCA2 mutation in the family. My sister and I both tested positive, and one day before her 40th birthday, she too was diagnosed with breast cancer. She urged me to have prophylactic surgery. At 37, I had bilateral mastectomies almost joyously, thinking I could relax about cancer. I desperately wanted a second child, but I couldn't conceive, and after much consideration, I decided to have an oophorectomy. My surgeon wasn't worried about my risk because of my young age; I felt it was too great. After the procedure, he said everything appeared normal and that 99 percent of pathology results came back clear. I rebounded quickly and was shopping when I received the call with my final pathology report—I cried and shook as I copied the information: "serous intra-epithelial tubal carcinoma, stage 0 in both fallopian tubes." I had cancer. It was caught before it could become invasive, and I required no further treatment. My diagnosis helped me find peace with my decision not to have that second child. My father had to develop breast cancer to save my life and my sister's. I know how lucky I am to be alive. —KISARIA*

The Importance of Clinical Trials

Clinical trials use human volunteers to determine whether new treatments work more effectively and safely than current standards. These well-designed, strictly controlled studies are the best way to advance breast and ovarian cancer care. Trials focus on screening, prevention, treatment, and quality of life. In phase 1 trials, an experimental drug or intervention is tested for the first time in a small group of people. Test results focus on safety, side effects, and dosage frequency and amount. The next step is a phase 2 trial to evaluate effectiveness and safety in a larger group, up to three hundred participants. Phase 3 trials compare the new treatment to the standard of care among thousands of people. Finally, phase 4 trials evaluate long-term side effects if the FDA approves a medication.

Clinical trials are necessary—improved treatments aren't possible without them—yet they can be conducted only when they recruit enough participants. Less than 5 percent of adult cancer patients participate. Clinical trials are particularly important for the BRCA community, which is much smaller than the general population. It's the only way we'll come to identify and understand the nuances of BRCA-related disease. If you take part in a clinical trial, you'll be monitored closely for any sign of disease progression. If your cancer doesn't respond to the trial drug, your participation will end, and you'll be offered another standard treatment or participation in a different clinical trial if you qualify. While some people fear they'll receive a placebo or an ineffective treatment, a placebo is used only when there is no standard-of-care treatment. You can get all this information and answers to any questions before agreeing to participate.

INSURANCE AND PAYMENT ISSUES

Treating cancer comes with a high price tag—it's a sad but true fact that many survivors don't discover until they're diagnosed. The Affordable Care Act of 2010 makes sweeping pro-patient changes to our health system over several years, with significant improvements to support and protect the healthcare needs of people who are genetically predisposed or diagnosed with cancer. Insurance companies may no longer refuse coverage; increase copays, deductibles, or premiums; or impose lifetime or annual dollar limits on essential benefits because you have cancer or a pre-existing condition. Preventive care, including mammograms, other routine screenings, and genetic counseling must be included in healthcare coverage at no extra cost. If your employer doesn't offer insurance, you can purchase health coverage from an exchange. You can view all scheduled changes from this legislation, including some that are already in effect, and implementation dates online at HealthCare.gov (www.healthcare.gov/law/timeline/index.html).

Effective 2014, federal law will require new insurance plans to cover participation in a clinical trial for cancer or other life-threatening illness and provide normal health care during your participation.

If you're disabled because of your cancer and your disability is expected to last for one year or more, you may be eligible for Social Security disability income benefits. Apply as soon as you become disabled—it can take up to six months before your request is approved and you begin receiving checks. Effective 2012, the Community Living Assistance Services and Supports Act provides affordable long-term home-care insurance. Medicare, Medicaid, and most healthcare and long-term insurers cover hospice services either in a facility or at home. Eligibility criteria and the extent of coverage and benefits varies depending on the individual policy; coverage usually includes medical equipment, medications, and nursing services. Some policies have a lifetime cap on hospice services, so be sure you understand what a policy covers before you purchase it. If you're uninsured or your plan doesn't cover hospice, ask your oncologist about facilities that will develop a payment plan or provide financial assistance.

THE FORCE PERSPECTIVE: WHEN CANCER IS FOUND DURING PROPHYLACTIC SURGERY

Although the goal of prophylactic surgery is to prevent cancer, sometimes that's when a tumor is discovered. If this happens to you, you're not alone. One study showed that 2.5 percent of BRCA mutation carriers who have prophylactic surgery already have ovarian cancer at the time of their operation.[8] As your healthcare team stages your disease and considers your best course of treatment, give yourself time to adjust to your diagnosis. Being diagnosed with cancer as you were taking steps to prevent it can be disheartening, even if you're grateful the cancer was discovered early. Treatment may shift your preventive timeline. If you're diagnosed with breast cancer, you might need to reschedule your oophorectomy or delay the reconstruction procedure you were planning. Be patient and kind with yourself. Try not to second-guess your decisions. Without a crystal ball, there's no way to foresee a diagnosis that seems to come out of the blue. Gather your resources, select a trusted healthcare team, and rally your support system around you. Do your homework and develop a plan of action, just as you did when you decided to be tested, and when you made your decisions about prophylactic surgery. You'll get through this and move forward.

WHAT TO REMEMBER ABOUT A DIAGNOSIS

- Your treatment decisions may be different from those of other women who are diagnosed but are not genetically predisposed to cancer.
- Once diagnosed, you may be at high risk for a new cancer.
- Genetics experts can help define your risk and develop a risk management plan for screening and prevention of future cancers.
- You can no longer be denied health insurance or have increased copays or deductibles solely because you're a previvor or a survivor.

LEARN MORE ABOUT DEALING WITH A DIAGNOSIS

Volumes of helpful information and resources are available to help you understand your diagnosis and treatment. Visit your library or bookstore or look online. Check the FORCE website for a list of special clinics that have a multidisciplinary approach to managing high-risk patients.

Cancer Care (www.cancercare.org) offers free support services for a variety of cancers.

Cancer Support Community (www.thewellnesscommunity.org) provides online resources, information, and local support affiliates.

Cancer Legal Resource Center (www.cancerlegalresourcecenter.org) provides free information and resources on cancer-related legal issues.

Clinicaltrials.gov gives information about clinical trials in the United States and around the world.

Chapter 19   Putting the Pieces

Together to Make

Difficult Decisions

You climb a mountain, edging slowly upwards.
Rock by rock,
step by step, one at a time.
From one point to another up the mountain.
From one height achieved to another.
—ANONYMOUS

KNOWING YOU'RE PREDISPOSED TO CANCER may not make your decisions easier, because without ideal ways to prevent or cure it, our current options are imperfect. Take your risk seriously, yet understand you can do something about it. Consider the short- and long-term outcomes for each alternative, and realize that your future decisions may be different from the ones you make now.

Deciding what to do can be agonizing. Is reliable early detection for ovarian cancer just a year away? Can you afford to wait to have your ovaries removed? Making complex decisions like these may seem like choosing the lesser of two (or three or four) evils. Even though you probably prefer none of them, knowing all your options allows you to consider each and choose the one that is best for you. While you may feel a sense of urgency to make a choice, you may also be fearful to proceed. How do you weigh all the options and consequences and choose effective decisions that you can live with? You do it one step at a time.

Start at the Beginning: Should You Be Tested?

Influenced by their family history, some people want to be tested for a BRCA mutation immediately. Others don't. If you're a candidate for genetic testing, but your fear of a positive result is holding you back, remember that many people test negative. And although facing the implications of a positive test is difficult, it provides the opportunity to be proactive. Regardless of your initial feelings, it's important to base your decisions on credible and up-to-date information. Your first step should be a consultation with a qualified genetics expert.

Making Decisions to Reduce Your Risk

Your priorities and tolerance for risk shape your decisions, which may not be the same as someone else in your situation. If you're a previvor in your twenties who wants to become pregnant within two years, you might choose preventive mastectomy before your pregnancy, particularly if you've seen young-onset breast cancer in your family. It not only reduces your risk, it eliminates the need for surveillance during pregnancy. If you feel strongly about breastfeeding, you may prefer surveillance. Whether you're a previvor or survivor, whatever you decide must be right for you. As you weigh your alternatives, you'll want to address two important outcomes: risk reduction and long-term survival.

Addressing Survival

If you have a BRCA mutation, breast and ovarian cancer pose a double threat. A Stanford University mathematical model projects how surveillance and preventive surgery affect survival in previvors. The model doesn't assume that one option provides better quality of life than another (for example, preventive mastectomy versus breast surveillance), since that's a subjective measurement. Instead, it offers information about the likely outcomes of both strategies, allowing women to rank options according to their own values. Chemoprevention alternatives aren't included in this analysis, because no conclusive evidence shows they affect life expectancy. The model does address the impact of young menopause (heart disease, osteoporosis/fractures, and dementia) on the risk of dying. The model doesn't assume routine use of hormone therapy after menopause, which might change the estimated benefit from preventive surgeries, or the impact of early menopause on survival (see table 20).

According to the model, mastectomy at age 25 and oophorectomy at age 40 lead to the greatest survival gains for carriers of a BRCA1 mutation. Increased breast surveillance (mammography and MRI screenings every year) combined with oophorectomy produces somewhat lower but similar results, because most breast cancers would likely be caught early enough to be treated successfully. The single most effective action is oophorectomy at or before age 40. Without any intervention, survival is projected to be considerably lower than for women in the general population.

If you have a mutation in BRCA2, survival estimates are more favorable,

Table 20. Effects of projected risk-reducing interventions

Intervention strategy	Probability of surviving to age 70 (%)
General population	84
BRCA1	
No intervention	53
Surveillance, no surgical intervention	59
PBM at 25, no oophorectomy	66
Oophorectomy at age 40	68
PBM at 25, oophorectomy at age 40	79
PBM at 40,* oophorectomy at age 40	77
Surveillance, oophorectomy at age 40	74
BRCA2	
No intervention	71
Surveillance, no surgical intervention	75
PBM at 25, no oophorectomy	79
PBM at 25, oophorectomy at age 40	83
PBM at 40,* oophorectomy at age 50	83
Surveillance, oophorectomy at age 40	80
Surveillance, oophorectomy at age 50	79

Source: Kurian AW, Sigal BM, Plevritis SK, "Survival Analysis of Cancer Risk Reduction Strategies for BRCA1/2 Mutation Carriers," *Journal of Clinical Oncology* 28, no. 2 (2010): 222–31.

* Includes screening with MRI and mammogram from ages 25 to 40

because your risk of gynecologic cancers is lower than that of someone with a BRCA1 mutation. Mastectomy at age 25 and oophorectomy at age 40 bring your estimated risk almost to the level of women who don't have a mutation. The model predicts a similar probability of survival for BRCA2 mutation carriers who delay mastectomy from age 25 until age 40 and delay oophorectomy from age 40 until age 50, because of the relatively low ovarian cancer risk they have before age 50.

Statistics help us make decisions; they don't guarantee the future. Your own survival outcome may be better or worse than these predictions. For now, the model is the most sophisticated survival tool available. It estimates cancer and survival in BRCA mutation carriers based on different strategies and may be helpful in your overall decision making, but keep in mind what it doesn't do. It doesn't factor in complex variables that might affect mortality or quality of life in people with BRCA mutations. Delaying preventive actions significantly affects your likelihood of being diagnosed with cancer.

Preventing Breast Cancer

People often make risk-reducing decisions based on whether a particular action will decrease their risk of dying from cancer. That's certainly important and something we're all very interested in. If you're at high risk for hereditary cancer, you may be equally concerned about avoiding diagnosis and treatment and how your risk-reducing decisions may affect your quality of life. If you'd rather avoid radiation or chemotherapy to treat breast cancer, even though you're likely to survive (as most women do), you may want to consider preventive mastectomy—it most effectively lowers the risk for a breast cancer diagnosis.

Comparing Your Options

As you weigh the options before you, use table 21 to consider ways to manage your risk. List additional advantages and disadvantages of these alternatives that affect you. Every concern you have is valid, no matter how small. You might be interested in a particular breast reconstructive

Table 21. Comparing risk-reducing alternatives

Action	Benefit	Limitation/risk
Surveillance for breast cancer	Increases odds of finding early stage cancer. Is less drastic than surgery.	Doesn't prevent or find all cancers. May detect benign abnormalities that require biopsy or additional tests. May cause anxiety about the screening or biopsies.
Surveillance for ovarian cancer	Is only slightly better than doing nothing.	Doesn't prevent cancer. May not improve odds of catching early stage cancer.
Chemoprevention for breast cancer	Reduces risk, but substantial risk remains. Tamoxifen and raloxifene may more effectively prevent ER+/PR+ breast cancers.	Doesn't guarantee you won't develop cancer. May cause menopause-like symptoms. Still requires close surveillance.
Mastectomy	Reduces breast cancer risk most effectively.	Loss of breasts and ability to breastfeed. Doesn't completely eliminate breast cancer risk. Not yet proven to improve survival.
Oral contraceptives	Reduces ovarian cancer risk by about 50%.	May increase breast cancer risk if used at a young age or for more than five years.
Oophorectomy (BSO)	Reduces risk for breast, ovarian, and fallopian tube cancers. Increases survival.	Small risk for primary peritoneal cancer remains. Causes immediate menopause and eliminates ability to conceive.

Table 22. Comparing treatment alternatives

Action	Benefit	Limitation/risk
Lumpectomy and radiation	Reduces risk of recurrence.	Doesn't reduce high risk for another primary diagnosis. May have to endure several weeks of radiation.
Unilateral mastectomy	Reduces risk in removed breast.	Doesn't address high risk in remaining breast.
Bilateral mastectomy	Almost completely removes future risk in both breasts.	Loss of breasts. May involve more extensive surgery and recuperation.
Oophorectomy (BSO)	Almost completely eliminates risk for ovarian and fallopian tube cancer. May improve prognosis.	Loss of fertility. Causes early menopause if you haven't entered natural menopause.

procedure for which you must travel to another city. That choice may represent a definite disadvantage if you can't afford the associated expense or have no one to care for your children when you're away or recovering. Work your way through all of your options, one by one, and be sure to discuss the medical benefits and risks with your healthcare team to ensure you've considered all possibilities. Then prioritize the list, eliminating unacceptable actions (see table 22).

Making Decisions about Treatment

Even two women with the same diagnosis may make different decisions about genetic testing and surgery. Diagnosed with breast cancer, one may feel it's wiser to be tested before surgery; that way, if she has a BRCA mutation, she might choose bilateral mastectomy to address her risk for a future breast cancer. If her test result is negative, she might proceed with a lumpectomy. A second woman, fearing even a week's delay in treatment, may decide to forego genetic testing and have a lumpectomy as quickly as possible rather than delaying surgery to wait for BRCA test results.

From Confused to Clear in Fifteen Steps

Genetic testing. Cancer risk. Preventive medications and surgeries. Fertility. These issues can be overwhelming, and you may think there's no light at the end of the tunnel. The key is to create order when your life may seem to be spinning out of control. Then that light will seem brighter and a lot more attainable.

1. Assemble your healthcare team, making sure each member is aware of what the others recommend.
2. Keep an organized binder of all your medical records, test results, research, and documents related to your previvor or survivor status.
3. Learn all you can about your absolute and relative risk, high-risk status, risk management options, or diagnosis and treatment alternatives.
4. Write down your questions and get answers.
5. Know when to stop researching: when you have all the information you can absorb and need to decide.
6. Recruit your family or friends to help research and provide a fresh perspective.
7. Allow yourself time to let it all sink in.
8. Give yourself a break. Take time to get away from information overload.
9. Take care of yourself. Eat balanced meals and get some physical activity most days.
10. Weigh the benefits and limitations of choosing or rejecting each option.
11. Consult the most knowledgeable professionals you can find for each decision.
12. Make your risk management or treatment decisions.
13. Cry or vent if you need to. (It's okay!)
14. Speak with a mental healthcare professional if you need help dealing with emotional stress.
15. Share. You don't have to face these issues alone. Reach out anytime to

FORCE in a way that is most comfortable for you: online (www.facing
ourrisk.org), through our helpline (866-288-7475), or in person at
your local FORCE outreach group. We can help put you in touch with
someone who went through similar decisions based on age, childbearing, cancer diagnosis, and other factors like your own.

MY STORY: My Family's Decisions

*At 32, my only sister developed early stage breast cancer with no lymph node
involvement. With no family history of breast cancer, we thought her diagnosis was an anomaly. Her medical team considered a double mastectomy
to be too radical for someone so young, so she had lumpectomy, radiation,
and chemotherapy. Nine months later, a new primary cancer appeared in her
other breast. This time it was in her lymph nodes. Within months, it spread
to her lungs, bones, and brain. Her oncologist said genetic testing wouldn't
change her treatment. He didn't consider whether it would affect me or other
female relatives, and he never recommended a genetic counselor. My sister
passed away, leaving her 4-year-old child without a mother.*

*Terrified about my own health, I rejoiced when my BRCA test result was
negative. My celebration was short-lived when I learned that a negative test
means little when there is no known familial mutation. My anxiety soared
out of control. I bruised myself looking for breast lumps, and I needed antidepressants to get through the days. Then I decided not to duplicate my sister's
experience. I learned about prophylactic mastectomy and oophorectomy and
contacted doctors. Finally, through FORCE, I was advised to see a genetic
counselor. I insisted we had no history of breast or ovarian cancer: my mother,
her two sisters, and their mother were alive and well. My father's only sister
and her daughters were too. The only cancer casualties were my paternal
great-grandmother (unknown young-onset cancer) and grandmother ("stomach cancer"). My counselor explained that the "stomach cancer" could have
been ovarian cancer and showed how a mutation could have passed from my
father to my sister without affecting other female relatives. She urged me to
have my parents tested. I left feeling scared, yet also empowered that my uninformative test could be informative if either parent tested positive.*

(continued)

Approaching my parents about testing was one of the hardest things I've ever done. They had lost their oldest child and wanted to put cancer behind them. It was unbearable for them to think that one of them might have passed the mutation to my sister that took her life. They wanted me to stop worrying. I couldn't. Eventually, they agreed, only if I alone received their results and never told them. One of them did test positive for a BRCA1 mutation, confirming me as a true negative. I didn't have prophylactic surgeries that year, but instead I delivered beautiful twin boys. —RHONDA

THE FORCE PERSPECTIVE: COPING WITH DECISIONS

Hereditary cancer doesn't end with a decision. Each answer, test result, and choice means sacrifices, and every sacrifice requires adjustment. You move forward step by step; each one requires emotional investment, usually followed with a period of grieving, accepting uncertainty, and adjusting to changes. No matter which course of action you choose, you must live with the consequences, whether or not things go according to plan. At some point, moving forward becomes a leap of faith that you've gathered as much information as you need, you know what to expect from the actions you decide upon, and you've chosen the best path forward. If the unexpected occurs—as it sometimes does—be patient and forgiving with yourself, and know that you made the best decision you could at the time. Then move on to the next set of decisions and deal with what lies ahead. In this way, we move forward and eventually allow ourselves to find joy in life and live it to the fullest.

WHAT TO REMEMBER ABOUT MAKING DECISIONS

- Consider strategies to manage both breast and ovarian cancer risk.
- Increased surveillance is a valid risk management option.
- Listen to others, but ultimately, make your own decisions about what's best for you.
- Your choices may change over time.

Notes

CHAPTER 1. BREAST AND OVARIAN CANCER BASICS

1. John EM, Miron A, Gong G, et al., "Prevalence of Pathogenic BRCA1 Mutation Carriers in Five U.S. Racial/Ethnic Groups," *Journal of the American Medical Association* 298, no. 24 (2007): 2869–76; Malone KE, Daling JR, Doody DR, et al., "Prevalence and Predictors of BRCA1 and BRCA2 Mutations in a Population-Based Study of Breast Cancer in White and Black American Women Ages 35 to 64 Years," *Cancer Research* 66, no. 16 (2006): 8297–8308; Risch HA, McLaughlin JR, Cole DE, et al., "Prevalence and Penetrance of Germline BRCA1 and BRCA2 Mutations in a Population Series of 649 Women with Ovarian Cancer," *American Journal of Human Genetics* 68, no. 3 (2001): 700–710.

2. Callahan MJ, Crum CP, Medeiros F, et al., "Primary Fallopian Tube Malignancies in BRCA-Positive Women Undergoing Surgery for Ovarian Cancer Risk Reduction," *Journal of Clinical Oncology* 25, no. 25 (2007): 3985–90.

3. Rebbeck TR, Kauff ND, Domchek SM, "Meta-analysis of Risk Reduction Estimates Associated with Risk-Reducing Salpingo-oophorectomy in BRCA1 or BRCA2 Mutation Carriers," *Journal of the National Cancer Institute* 101, no. 2 (2009): 80–87; Kauff ND, Domchek SM, Friebel TM, et al., "Risk-Reducing Salpingo-Oophorectomy for the Prevention of BRCA1- and BRCA2-Associated Breast and Gynecological Cancer. A Multicenter, Prospective Study," *Journal of Clinical Oncology* 26, no. 8 (2008): 1331–37.

4. Tersmette AC, Petersen GM, Offerhaus GJ, et al., "Increased Risk of Incident Pancreatic Cancer among First-Degree Relatives of Patients with Familial Pancreatic Cancer," *Clinical Cancer Research* 7, no. 3 (2001): 738–44.

5. Thompson D, Easton DF, and The Breast Cancer Linkage Consortium, "Cancer Incidence in BRCA1 Mutation Carriers," *Journal of the National Cancer Institute* 94, no. 18 (2002): 1358–1365; The Breast Cancer Linkage Consortium, "Cancer Risks in BRCA2 Mutation Carriers," *Journal of the National Cancer Institute* 91, no. 15 (1999): 1310–16.

6. The Breast Cancer Linkage Consortium, "Cancer Risks in BRCA2 Mutation Carriers," 1310–16.

CHAPTER 2. A PEEK INSIDE

1. Peto J, Collins N, Barfoot R, et al., "Prevalence of BRCA1 and BRCA2 Gene Mutations in Patients with Early Onset Breast Cancer," *Journal of the National Cancer Institute* 91, no. 11 (1999): 943–49; Whittemore AS, Gong G, John EM, et al., "Prevalence of BRCA1 Mutation Carriers Among U.S. Non-Hispanic Whites," *Cancer Epidemiology, Biomarkers & Prevention* 13, no. 12 (2004): 2078–83.

2. Kurian AW, "BRCA1 and BRCA2 Mutations Across Race and Ethnicity: Distribution and Clinical Implications," *Current Opinion in Obstetrics and Gynecology* 22, no. 1 (2010): 72–78; John EM, Miron A, Gong G, et al., "Prevalence of Pathogenic BRCA1 Mutation Carriers in Five U.S. Racial/Ethnic Groups," *Journal of the American Medical Association* 298, no. 24 (2007): 2869–76.

CHAPTER 3. DEFINING RISK

1. Collaborative Group on Hormonal Factors in Breast Cancer, "Familial Breast Cancer: Collaborative Reanalysis of Individual Data from 52 Epidemiological Studies Including 58,209 Women with Breast Cancer and 101,986 Women without the Disease," *Lancet* 358, no. 9291 (2001): 1389–99.

2. Kauff ND, Mitra N, Robson ME, et al., "Risk of Ovarian Cancer in BRCA1 and BRCA2 Mutation-Negative Hereditary Breast Cancer Families," *Journal of the National Cancer Institute* 97, no. 18 (2005): 1382–84.

3. Barnholtz-Sloan JS, Schwartz AG, Qureshi F, et al., "Ovarian Cancer: Changes in Patterns at Diagnosis and Relative Survival Over the Last Three Decades," *American Journal of Obstetrics & Gynecology* 189, no. 4 (2003): 1120–27.

CHAPTER 4. HEREDITARY CANCER

1. Eng C, "Cowden Syndrome and Related Disorders," *Familial Breast and Ovarian Cancer. Genetics, Screening and Management*, edited by Patrick J Morrison, Shirley V Hodgson, and Neva E Haites, 22–42. Cambridge, UK: Cambridge University Press, 2002.

2. Garber JE, Goldstein AM, Kantor AF, et al., "Follow-up Study of Twenty-four Families with Li-Fraumeni Syndrome," *Cancer Research* 51, no. 22 (1991): 6094–97.

3. Pharoah PD, Guilford P, Caldas C, "Incidence of Gastric Cancer and Breast Cancer in CDH1 (E-cadherin) Mutation Carriers from Hereditary Diffuse Gastric Cancer Families," *Gastroenterology* 121, no. 6 (2001): 1348–53; Kaurah P, MacMillan A, Boyd N, et al., "Founder and Recurrent CDH1 Mutations in Families with Hereditary Diffuse Gastric Cancer," *Journal of the American Medical Association* 297, no. 21 (2007): 2360–72.

4. Begg CB, Orlow I, Hummer AJ, et al., "Lifetime Risk of Melanoma in

CDKN2A Mutation Carriers in a Population-Based Sample," *Journal of the National Cancer Institute* 97, no. 20 (2005): 1507–15.

CHAPTER 6. GENETIC TESTING

1. Weitzel JN, Lagos VI, Cullinane CA, et al., "Limited Family Structure and BRCA Gene Mutation Status in Single Cases of Breast Cancer," *Journal of the American Medical Association* 297, no. 23 (2007): 2587–95.

CHAPTER 8. EARLY DETECTION STRATEGIES

1. Samphao S, Wheeler A, Rafferty E, et al., "Diagnosis of Breast Cancer in Women Age 40 and Younger: Delays in Diagnosis are Common Due to Underutilization of Genetic Testing and Breast Imaging," American Society of Breast Surgeons, presented at ASBS annual meeting, 2009.

2. Wilke L, Broadwater G, Rabiner S, et al., "Breast Self-Examination: Defining a Cohort Still in Need," American Society of Breast Surgeons, poster presentation at ASBS annual meeting, 2009.

3. Pisano E, Gatsonis C, Hendrick E, et al., "Diagnostic Performance of Digital versus Film Mammography for Breast Cancer Screening—The Results of the American College of Radiology Imaging Network (ACRIN) Digital Mammographic Imaging Screening Trial (DMIST)," *New England Journal of Medicine* 353, no. 17 (2005): 1773–83.

4. Berrington de Gonzalez A, Berg CD, Visvanathan K, et al., "Estimated Risk of Radiation-Induced Breast Cancer from Mammographic Screening for Young BRCA Mutation Carriers," *Journal of the National Cancer Institute* 101, no. 3 (2009): 205–209.

5. Kagay CR, Quale C, and Smith-Bindman R, "Screening Mammography in the American Elderly," *American Journal of Preventive Medicine* 31, no. 2 (2006): 142–49.

6. Lord SJ, Lei W, Craft P, et al., "A Systematic Review of the Effectiveness of Magnetic Resonance Imaging (MRI) as an Addition to Mammography and Ultrasound in Screening Young Women at High Risk of Breast Cancer," *European Journal of Cancer* 43, no. 13 (2007): 1905–17.

7. Fishman DA, Cohen L, Blank S, et al., "The Role of Ultrasound Evaluation in the Detection of Early Stage Epithelial Ovarian Cancer," *American Journal of Obstetrics & Gynecology* 192, no. 4 (2005): 1214–21.

8. Ovarian Cancer National Alliance, "Detection," www.ovariancancer.org /about-ovarian-cancer/detection.

9. Chan JK, Kapp DS, Shin JY, et al., "Influence of the Gynecologic Oncologist on the Survival of Ovarian Cancer Patients," *Obstetrics & Gynecology* 109, no. 6 (2007): 1342–50.

CHAPTER 9. CHEMOPREVENTION

1. Metcalfe K, Lynch HT, Ghadirian P, et al., "Contralateral Breast Cancer in BRCA1 and BRCA2 Mutation Carriers," *Journal of Clinical Oncology* 22, no. 12 (2004): 2328–35.

2. King MC, Wieand S, Hale K, et al., National Surgical Adjuvant Breast and Bowel Project (NSABP-P1) Breast Cancer Prevention Trial, "Tamoxifen and Breast Cancer Incidence Among Women with Inherited Mutations in BRCA1 and BRCA2," *Journal of the American Medical Association* 286, no. 18 (2001): 2251–56.

3. Powles TJ, Ashley S, Tidy A, et al., "Twenty-Year Follow-up of the Royal Marsden Randomized, Double-Blinded Tamoxifen Breast Cancer Prevention Trial," *Journal of the National Cancer Institute* 99, no. 4 (2007): 283–90.

4. Ibid.

5. Howell A, Cuzick J, Baum M, et al., ATAC Trialists' Group, "Results of the ATAC (Arimidex, Tamoxifen, Alone or in Combination) Trial After Completion of 5 years' Adjuvant Treatment for Breast Cancer," *Lancet* 365, no. 9453 (2005): 60–62.

6. Harris RE, Chlebowski RT, Jackson RD, et al., "Breast Cancer and Nonsteroidal Anti-Inflammatory Drugs Prospective Results from the Women's Health Initiative," *Cancer Research* 63 (2003): 6096.

7. Eliassen AH, Chen WY, Spiegelman D, et al., "Use of Aspirin, Other Nonsteroidal Anti-Inflammatory Drugs, and Acetaminophen and Risk of Breast Cancer Among Premenopausal Women in the Nurses' Health Study II," *Archives of Internal Medicine* 169 (2009): 115–21.

8. Solomon SD, McMurray JJ, Pfeffer MA, et al., "Cardiovascular Risk Associated with Celecoxib in a Clinical Trial for Colorectal Adenoma Prevention," *New England Journal of Medicine* 352 (2005): 1071–80.

9. Veronesi U, Mariani L, Decensi A, et al., "Fifteen-Year Results of a Randomized Phase III Trial of Fenretinide to Prevent Second Breast Cancer," *Annals of Oncology* 17, no. 7 (2006): 1065–71.

10. Kochhar R, Khurana V, Bejjanki H, et al., "Statins Reduce Breast Cancer Risk: A Case Control Study in U.S. Female Veterans," Presented at American Society of Clinical Oncologists, 2005. Abstract 514.

11. Chlebowski RT, Chen Z, Cauley JA, et al., "Oral Bisphosphonate Use and Breast Cancer Incidence in Postmenopausal Women," *Journal of Clinical Oncology* 28, no. 22 (2010): 3582–90.

12. Rennert G, Pinchev M, Rennert HS, "Use of Bisphosphonates and Risk of Postmenopausal Breast Cancer," *Journal of Clinical Oncology* 28, no. 22 (2010): 3577–81.

13. Bodmer M, Meier C, Krähenbühl S, et al., "Long-term Metformin Use Is Associated with Decreased Risk of Breast Cancer," *Diabetes Care* 33, no. 6 (2010): 1304–1308.

14. Modan B, Hartge P, Hirsh-Yechezkel G, et al., "Parity, Oral Contraceptives,

and the Risk of Ovarian Cancer among Carriers and Noncarriers of a BRCA1 or BRCA2 Mutation," *New England Journal of Medicine* 345, no. 4 (2001): 235–40.

15. De Palo G, Mariani L, Camerini T, et al., "Effect of Fenretinide on Ovarian Carcinoma Occurrence," *Gynecologic Oncology* 86, no. 1 (2002): 24–27.

CHAPTER 10. MASTECTOMY FOR RISK REDUCTION AND TREATMENT

1. Rebbeck TR, Friebel T, Lynch HT, et al., "Bilateral Prophylactic Mastectomy Reduces Breast Cancer Risk in BRCA1 and BRCA2 Mutation Carriers: The PROSE Study Group," *Journal of Clinical Oncology* 22, no. 6 (2004): 1055–62.

2. Pierce L, Phillips K, Griffith K, et al., "Local Therapy Options in BRCA1/2 Carriers with Operable Breast Cancer: The Importance of Adjuvant Chemotherapy," *European Journal of Cancer* 8, no. 3 (2010): 55.

3. Seynaeve C, Verhoog LC, van de Bosch LM, et al., "Ipsilateral Breast Tumour Recurrence in Hereditary Breast Cancer Following Breast-Conserving Therapy," *European Journal of Cancer* 40, no. 8 (2004): 1150–58.

4. Pierce L, et al., "Local Therapy Options," 55.

5. Tuttle TM, Habermann EB, Grund EH, et al., "Increasing Use of Contra-lateral Prophylactic Mastectomy for Breast Cancer Patients: A Trend Toward More Aggressive Surgical Treatment," *Journal of Clinical Oncology* 25, no. 33 (2007): 5203–5209.

6. Malone KF, Begg CB, Haile RW, et al., "Population-Based Study of the Risk of Second Primary Contralateral Breast Cancer Associated with Carrying a Muta-tion in BRCA1 or BRCA2," *Journal of Clinical Oncology* 28, no. 14 (2010): 2404–2410.

7. Sorbero ME, Dick AW, Beckjord EB, et al., "Diagnostic Breast Magnetic Resonance Imaging and Contralateral Prophylactic Mastectomy," *Annals of Surgical Oncology* 16, no. 6 (2009): 1597–1605.

CHAPTER 11. RECONSTRUCTION

1. American Society of Plastic Surgeons, "2009 Reconstructive Surgery Trends," (www.plasticsurgery.org/News-and-Resources.html).

CHAPTER 12. OOPHORECTOMY AND OTHER RISK-REDUCING GYNECOLOGIC SURGERIES

1. Rebbeck TR, Lynch HT, Neuhausen SL, et al., "Prophylactic Oophorectomy in Carriers of BRCA1 or BRCA2 Mutations," *New England Journal of Medicine* 346, no. 21 (2002): 1616–22; Berek JS, Chalas E, Edelson M, et al., "Prophylactic and Risk-Reducing Bilateral Salpingo-Oophorectomy. Recommendations Based on Risk of Ovarian Cancer," *Obstetrics & Gynecology* 116, no. 3 (2010): 733–43; Grann

VR, Jacobson JS, Thomason D, et al., "Effect of Prevention Strategies on Survival and Quality-Adjusted Survival of Women with BRCA1/2 Mutations: An Updated Decision Analysis," *Journal of Clinical Oncology* 20, no. 10 (2002): 2520–29; Kauff ND, Satagopan JM, Robson ME, et al., "Risk-Reducing Salpingo-oophorectomy in Women with a *BRCA1* or *BRCA2* Mutation," *New England Journal of Medicine* 346, no. 21 (2002): 1609–15.

2. Rebbeck TR, et al., "Prophylactic Oophorectomy," 1616–22.

3. Metcalfe K, Lynch HT, Ghadirian P, et al., "Contralateral Breast Cancer in BRCA1 and BRCA2 Mutation Carriers," *Journal of Clinical Oncology* 22, no. 12 (2004): 2328–35.

4. Rebbeck TR, Kauff ND, Domchek SM, "Meta-analysis of Risk Reduction Estimates Associated with Risk-Reducing Salpingo-oophorectomy in BRCA1 or BRCA2 Mutation Carriers," *Journal of the National Cancer Institute* 101, no. 2 (2009): 80–87; Kauff ND, Domchek SM, Friebel TM, et al., "Risk-Reducing Salpingo-Oophorectomy for the Prevention of BRCA1- and BRCA2-Associated Breast and Gynecological Cancer: A Multicenter, Prospective Study," *Journal of Clinical Oncology* 26, no. 8 (2008): 1331–37.

5. Powell CB, Kenley E, Chen LM, et al., "Risk-Reducing Salpingo-Oophorectomy in BRCA Mutation Carriers: Role of Serial Sectioning in the Detection of Occult Malignancy," *Journal of Clinical Oncology* 23, no. 1 (2005): 127–32.

CHAPTER 13. DEALING WITH MENOPAUSE AND QUALITY-OF-LIFE ISSUES

1. Modell JG, May RS, Katholi CR, "Effect of Bupropion-SR on Orgasmic Dysfunction in Nondepressed Subjects: A Pilot Study," *Journal of Sex & Marital Therapy* 26, no. 3 (2000): 231–40.

2. Mathias C, Cardeal Mendes CM, Pondé de Sena E, et al., "An Open-Label, Fixed-Dose Study of Bupropion Effect on Sexual Function Scores in Women Treated for Breast Cancer," *Annals of Oncology* 17, no. 12 (2006): 1792–96.

3. Caan B, Neuhouser M, Aragaki A, et al., "Calcium Plus Vitamin D Supplementation and the Risk of Postmenopausal Weight Gain," *Archives of Internal Medicine* 167, no. 9 (2007): 893–902.

4. Shuster LT, Gostout BS, Grossardt BR, et al., "Prophylactic Oophorectomy in Pre-Menopausal Women and Long-Term Health—A Review," *Menopause International* 14, no. 3 (2008): 111–16.

5. National Osteoporosis Foundation, "Fast Facts," www.nof.org/node/40.

6. Rebbeck TR, Friebel T, Wagner T, et al., "Effect of Short-Term Hormone Replacement Therapy on Breast Cancer Risk Reduction after Bilateral Prophylactic Oophorectomy in BRCA1 and BRCA2 Mutation Carriers: The PROSE Study Group," *Journal of Clinical Oncology* 23, no. 31 (2005): 7804–7810.

7. Ibid.

8. Writing Group for the Women's Health Initiative Investigators, "Risks and Benefits of Estrogen Plus Progestin in Healthy Postmenopausal Women: Principal Results from the Women's Health Initiative Randomized Controlled Trial," *Journal of the American Medical Association* 288, no. 3 (2002): 321–33; Stefanick ML, Anderson GL, Margolis KL, et al., "Effects of Conjugated Equine Estrogens on Breast Cancer and Mammography Screening in Postmenopausal Women with Hysterectomy," *Journal of the American Medical Association* 295, no. 14 (2006): 1647–57.

9. U.S. Food and Drug Administration, "Report: Limited FDA Survey of Compounded Drug Products," www.fda.gov/Drugs/GuidanceComplianceRegulatory Information/PharmacyCompounding/ucm155725.htm.

10. Holmberg L and Anderson H for the HABITS steering and data safety monitoring committees, "HABITS (Hormonal Replacement Therapy after Breast Cancer—Is It Safe?), a Randomised Comparison: Trial Stopped," *Lancet* 363, no. 9407 (2004): 453–55.

CHAPTER 14. MANAGING LIFESTYLE CHOICES

1. Brasky TM, Lampe JW, Potter JD, et al., "Specialty Supplements and Breast Cancer Risk in the VITamins And Lifestyle (VITAL) Cohort," *Cancer Epidemiology, Biomarkers & Prevention* 19, no. 7 (2010): 1696–1708.

2. Georgetown University Medical Center, "News Release: Breast Cancer Risk Tied to Grandmother's Diet," *Science Daily*, April 20, 2010, http://explore.george town.edu/news/?ID=50223&PageTemplateID=295.

3. Linos E, Willett WC, Cho E, et al., "Adolescent Diet in Relation to Breast Cancer Risk Among Premenopausal Women," *Cancer Epidemiology, Biomarkers & Prevention* 19, no. 3 (2010): 689–96.

4. Ghadirian P, Narod SA, Farfard E, et al., "Breast Cancer Risk in Relation to the Joint Effect of BRCA Mutations and Diet Diversity," *Breast Cancer Research and Treatment* 117, no. 2 (2009): 417–22.

5. Buck K, Zaineddin AK, Vrieling A, et al., "Meta-Analyses of Lignans and Enterolignans in Relation to Breast Cancer Risk," *American Journal of Clinical Nutrition* 92, no. 1 (2010): 141–53.

6. Frazier AL, Ryan CT, Rockett H, et al., "Adolescent Diet and Risk of Breast Cancer," *Breast Cancer Research* 5, no. 3 (2003): R59–R64.

7. Brasky TM, et al., "Specialty Supplements," 1696.

8. U.S. Department of Health and Human Services, "The Surgeon General's Call to Action to Prevent and Decrease Overweight and Obesity," www.surgeon general.gov/topics/obesity/calltoaction/fact_adolescents.htm.

9. American Institute for Cancer Research, "Landmark Report: Excess Body Fat Causes Cancer," www.aicr.org/site/News2?page=NewsArticle&id=12898&news _iv_ctrl=0&abbr=pr_.

10. Leitzmann MF, Koebnick C, Danforth KN, et al., "Body Mass Index and Risk of Ovarian Cancer," *Cancer* 115, no. 4 (2009): 812–22.

11. King MC, Marks JH, and Mandell JB, New York Breast Cancer Study Group, "Breast and Ovarian Cancer Risks Due to Inherited Mutations in BRCA1 and BRCA2," *Science* 302, no. 5645 (2003): 643–46.

12. Kotsopoulos J, Olopade OI, Ghadirian P, et al., "Changes in Body Weight and the Risk of Breast Cancer in BRCA1 and BRCA2 Mutation Carriers," *Breast Cancer Research* 7, no. 5 (2005): R833–R843.

13. King MC, et al., "Breast and Ovarian Cancer Risks," 643–46.

14. Eisen A, Lubinski J, Gronwald J, et al., and the Hereditary Breast Cancer Clinical Study Group, "Hormone Therapy and the Risk of Breast Cancer in BRCA1 Mutation Carriers," *Journal of the National Cancer Institute* 100, no. 19 (2008): 1361–67.

15. Mørch LS, Løkkegaard E, Andreasen AH, et al., "Hormone Therapy and Ovarian Cancer," *Journal of the American Medical Association* 302, no. 3 (2009): 298–305.

16. Collishaw NE, Boyd NF, Cantor KP, et al., and the Ontario Tobacco Research Unit, "Canadian Expert Panel on Tobacco Smoke and Breast Cancer Risk," 2009, www.otru.org/pdf/special/expert_panel_tobacco_breast_cancer.pdf.

17. Li CI, Daling JR, Porter PL, et al., "Relationship Between Potentially Modifiable Lifestyle Factors and Risk of Second Primary Contralateral Breast Cancer Among Women Diagnosed with Estrogen Receptor-Positive Invasive Breast Cancer," *Journal of Clinical Oncology* 27, no. 32 (2009): 5312–18.

CHAPTER 15. SHARING INFORMATION WITH FRIENDS, FAMILY, AND COWORKERS

1. Hoskins LM, Roy K, Peters JA, et al., "Disclosure of Positive BRCA1/2 Mutation Status in Young Couples: The Journey from Uncertainty to Bonding through Partner Support," *Families, Systems and Health* 26, no. 3 (2008): 296–316.

CHAPTER 16. YOUNG AND AT HIGH RISK

1. Young Survival Coalition, "Young Women and Breast Cancer," www.youngsurvival.org/young-women-and-bc/.

2. Samphao S, Wheeler A, Rafferty E, et al., "Diagnosis of Breast Cancer in Women Age 40 and Younger: Delays in Diagnosis are Common Due to Underutilization of Genetic Testing and Breast Imaging," presented at ASBS annual meeting, 2009.

3. Chetrit A, Hirsh-Yechezkel G, Ben-David Y, et al., "Effect of BRCA1/2 Mutations on Long-Term Survival of Patients with Invasive Ovarian Cancer: The National Israeli Study of Ovarian Cancer," *Journal of Clinical Oncology* 26, no. 1 (2008): 20–25.

4. American Cancer Society, "Lifestyle-Related Factors and Breast Cancer Risk, Recent Oral Contraceptive Use," www.cancer.org/Cancer/BreastCancer /DetailedGuide/breast-cancer-risk-factors.

5. Narod SA, Risch H, Moslehi R, et al., "Oral Contraceptives and the Risk of Hereditary Ovarian Cancer," *New England Journal of Medicine* 339 (1998): 424–28.

6. Quinn GP, Vadaparampil ST, Jacobsen P, et al., "National Survey of Physicians Practice Patterns: Fertility Preservation and Cancer Patients," *Journal of Clinical Oncology* 27, no. 35 (2009): 5952–57.

7. Jernström H, Lubinski J, Lynch H, et al., "Breast-Feeding and the Risk of Breast Cancer in BRCA1 and BRCA2 Mutation Carriers," *Journal of the National Cancer Institute* 96, no. 14 (2004): 1094–98.

8. Domchek SM, Friebel TM, Singer CF, et al., "Association of Risk-Reducing Surgery in BRCA1 or BRCA2 Mutation Carriers with Cancer Risk and Mortality," *Journal of the American Medical Association* 304, no. 9 (2010): 967–75; Rebbeck TR, Friebel T, Wagner T, et al., "Effect of Short-Term Hormone Replacement Therapy on Breast Cancer Risk Reduction after Bilateral Prophylactic Oophorectomy in BRCA1 and BRCA2 Mutation Carriers: The PROSE Study Group," *Journal of Clinical Oncology* 23, no. 31 (2005): 7804–10.

CHAPTER 17. HOW BRCA AFFECTS MEN

1. Basham VM, Lipscombe JM, Ward JM, et al., "BRCA1 and BRCA2 Mutations in a Population-Based Study of Male Breast Cancer," *Breast Cancer Research* 4, no. 1 (2002): R2.

2. Wisinski KB and Gradishar WJ. "Male Breast Cancer." *Diseases of the Breast*, edited by JR Harris, ME Lippman, CK Osborne and M Morrow, 775–80. Philadelphia: Lippincott, Williams & Wilkins, 2010.

3. Shao YH, Albertsen PC, Roberts CB, et al., "Risk Profiles and Treatment Patterns Among Men Diagnosed as Having Prostate Cancer and a Prostate-Specific Antigen Level Below 4.0 ng/ml," *Archives of Internal Medicine* 170, no. 14 (2010): 1256–61.

4. Mitra AV, Bancroft EK, Barbachano Y, et al., "Targeted Prostate Cancer Screening in Men with Mutations in BRCA1 and BRCA2 Detects Aggressive Prostate Cancer: Preliminary Analysis of the Results of the IMPACT Study," *British Journal of Urology International* (2010) Epub ahead of print. doi: 10.1111/j.146 4-410X.2010.09648.x.

5. Fong PC, Boss DS, Yap TA, et al., "Inhibition of Poly (ADP-Ribose) Polymerase in Tumors from BRCA Mutation Carriers," *New England Journal of Medicine* 361, no. 2 (2009): 123–34.

6. Augustsson K, Michaud DS, Rimm EB, et al., "A Prospective Study of Intake of Fish and Marine Fatty Acids and Prostate Cancer," *Cancer Epidemiology, Biomarkers & Prevention* 12, no 1 (2003): 64–67.

CHAPTER 18. DIAGNOSIS

1. Byrski T, Huzarski T, Dent R, et al., "Response to Neoadjuvant Therapy with Cisplatin in BRCA1-Positive Breast Cancer Patients," *Breast Cancer Research and Treatment* 115, no. 2 (2009): 359–63.

2. O'Shaughnessy J, et al., "Updated Results of a Randomized Phase II Study Demonstrating Efficacy and Safety of BS1-201, a PARP Inhibitor, in Combination with Gemcitabine/Carboplatin in Metastatic Triple-Negative Breast Cancer," San Antonio Breast Cancer Symposium, 2009. Abstract 3122.

3. Fong PC, Boss DS, Yap TA, et al., "Inhibition of Poly (ADP-Ribose) Polymerase in Tumors from BRCA Mutation Carriers," *New England Journal of Medicine* 361, no. 2 (2009): 123–34; Audeh MW, Penson RT, Friedlander M, et al., "Phase II Trial of the Oral PARP Inhibitor Olaparib (AZD2281) in BRCA-Deficient Advanced Ovarian Cancer," *Journal of Clinical Oncology* 27, no. 15s (2009): 5500.

4. Chetrit A, Hirsh-Yechezkel G, Ben-David Y, et al., "Effect of BRCA1/2 Mutations on Long-Term Survival of Patients with Invasive Ovarian Cancer: The National Israeli Study of Ovarian Cancer," *Journal of Clinical Oncology* 26, no. 1 (2008): 20–25.

5. Metcalfe KA, Lynch HT, Ghadirian P, et al., "The Risk of Ovarian Cancer after Breast Cancer in BRCA1 and BRCA2 Carriers," *Gynecologic Oncology* 96, no. 1 (2005): 222–26.

6. Metcalfe KA, et al., "The Risk of Ovarian Cancer," 222–26.

7. Kauff ND, Mitra N, Robson ME, et al., "Risk of Ovarian Cancer in BRCA1 and BRCA2 Mutation-Negative Hereditary Breast Cancer Families," *Journal of the National Cancer Institute* 97, no. 18 (2005): 1382–84.

8. Domchek SM, Friebel TM, Garber JE, et al., "Occult Ovarian Cancers Identified at Risk-Reducing Salpingo-Oophorectomy in a Prospective Cohort of BRCA1/2 Mutation Carriers," *Breast Cancer Research and Treatment* 124, no. 1 (2010): 195–203.

Index

f indicates a figure; t indicates a table

abdominal flap reconstruction, 128–29
abdominal wash, 140–41
abdominal weakness after TRAM, 129, 134
abortion and breast cancer risk, 18
absolute risk, defined, 31–32
acellular dermal matrix tissue, 126
Actonel, 102, 159
acupuncture, 118
adjuvant chemotherapy, 115, 218
adoption, 202
African Americans, risk and cancer rates, 7–8, 12, 29, 70
age, and breast cancer risk, 5–8, 23, 25–29, 31–33, 34t, 39t, 40–41, 62, 77–80, 99–101, 103–4
age, and ovarian cancer risk, 9, 23, 25, 28, 34t, 39t, 84t, 148. *See also* young women at high risk
alcohol consumption, 30, 153, 156, 164, 170, 208
alpha-linolenic acid, 174
alternative medicine, 162–63
American Cancer Society information: alcohol consumption as risk factor, 178; and donation of surgical services, 119; and finding specialists, 217; and high-risk criteria for breast cancer, 83; high-risk screening recommendations of, 78t; and menopause and uterine

cancer risk, 91; and obesity and ovarian cancer risk, 175; and PSA testing recommendations, 211
American Institute for Cancer Research, 171, 175–76
American Lung Association, 180
American Society of Clinical Oncology, 22, 199
American Society of Plastic Surgeons, 127
analgesics and ovarian cancer risk, 104
anaplastic large cell lymphoma, 124
anatomy: of breast, 5f; of female reproductive system, 8f
androgen deprivation therapy, 212
antidepressants, 96, 154
antioxidants, 174, 181
areolas, 110–12
areola-sparing mastectomy, 113–14
areola tattoos, 121, 131–32
aromatase inhibitors (AIs), 98–99, 147, 210
Ashkenazi Jews and BRCA mutation, 23, 37, 54, 59, 69
Asian Americans, risk and cancer rates, 29, 52, 172, 174
aspirin, 99–100, 154, 156
ataxia-telangiectasia (AT), 41
atrophied vaginal tissues, 152
attached flap reconstruction, 128–29
atypical ductal hyperplasia (ADH), 32–33

autologous breast reconstruction. *See* tissue flap reconstruction
average risk, 25, 33–34, 34*t*
axillary lymph node dissection. *See* sampling lymph nodes

benign growths, 40, 79, 82, 86, 88, 90, 196, 208
bilateral mastectomy. *See* mastectomy
bilateral salpingo-oophorectomy (BSO). *See* oophorectomy
bioidentical hormones, 162
biomarkers, for ovarian cancer, 86–87
biopsy: endometrial, 91; MRI-guided, 83–84; needle, 88; sentinel node, 109–10, 210; stereotactic, 89; surgical, 89. *See also* breast biopsy
birth control, 145, 150, 198
bisphenol A (BPA), 181
bisphosphonates, 101–2, 159, 210
black cohosh, 151
bladder prolapse, 144
blood clots, 97–98, 103, 160
blood-thinning medications, 154
body mass index (BMI), 175
bone density, 97–98
bone density tests, 158–59, 164
bone fractures, 102, 158
bone loss, menopausal, 158–59
Boniva, 102, 159
BRACAnalysis Rearrangement Test (BART), 59–60
BRACAnalysis test, 58–60, 63
brachytherapy, 212
BRCA1 gene mutation, overview: and average risk for carriers, 33, 34*t*; and breast cancer, 3–4, 8, 219; and breast-feeding to reduce breast cancer risk, 201; and contralateral breast cancer, 116; discovery of, 15; in men, 206*t*, 208*t*; and ovarian cancer, 3–4, 223; and pancreatic cancer, 12, 23; and

survival probability, 230–31, 230*t*; and tamoxifen, 54, 95, 99; and testing, 58–60; and triple-negative type breast cancers, 8. *See also specific aspects*
BRCA2 gene mutation, overview: and average risk for carriers, 33–34*t*; and breast cancer, 3–4, 8; and cancer-related hormone receptors, 7–8; and contralateral breast cancer, 116; discovery of, 15; and Fanconi anemia, 37; and melanoma, 12, 92, 180; in men, 206*t*, 208*t*, 211, 214; and ovarian cancer, 3–4, 223; and pancreatic cancer, 12, 23; and survival probability, 230–31; and tamoxifen, 95, 99; and testing, 58–60. *See also specific aspects*
BRCA genes, overview: and damage control process, 20; and family history risk, 23; function of, 18, 22; inheritability of, 36–37; and large rearrangements, 59
BRCA mutation, 4, 38; inherited from father, 36, 38; inherited from mother, 36, 38; and risk of other hereditary cancers, 38–42
breast anatomy, 5*f*
breast biopsy, 82–84, 88–89, 209; LCIS detection, 6; as risk factor, 29
breast cancer, overview: and atypical ductal hyperplasia, 32–33; and chemoprevention, 94–103; and comparison of risk-reducing methods, 232*t*; comparison of treatments for, 233*t*; early onset, 103–4; hereditary, defined, 27, 38–39, 115; incidence of, 3–7, 25–26, 217; in men, 207–10; and ovarian cancer risk, 223; and overexpression of HER2/neu, 8, 210; post-menopausal, 94–99, 169, 173–76; and pregnancy, 199–200; premenopausal, 6, 23, 80, 82–83, 95, 98, 100–101, 104, 147, 171, 173, 179; sporadic, defined,

3–4; and surveillance, 77–84, 89, 209; and triple-negative, 8, 29, 102, 219; and tumor characteristics, 6–8, 21; types of, 6–7. *See also specific types and treatments*

breast cancer risk: for average woman, 5, 25–26; lifetime, with BRCA mutation, 32–34; after mastectomy, 113; after ovarian cancer, 222; and risk factors, 28–31

breast density, 29, 83, 101, 195–96

breastfeeding, 198–201, 229

breast implants: acellular dermal matrix tissue, 126; capsular contracture, 127; comparison of techniques, 131*t*; direct-to-implant reconstruction, 125–26, 136; procedures, 124–26; and radiation therapy, 121–22; replacement of, 127; safety issues, 124; saline and silicone, 122, 124–27

breast MRI. *See* magnetic resonance imaging (MRI)

breast prostheses, 123

breast reconstruction, 121–37; adding nipples/areolas, 131–32; choosing a plastic surgeon, 121, 134–35, 137; and comparison of techniques, 131*t*; and cosmetic issues, 133; delayed, 121–22; with expanders, 122, 124–25, 131*t*; immediate, 108–10; with implants, 122, 124–27, 131*t*, 136; and insurance and payment issues, 135–36; for men, 209; and nipple projection, 133–34; and recovery, 121, 124–26, 129–34; and risks, 133*t*; and sensation, 108, 132; and symmetry, 116, 122, 134; with tissue flaps, 122, 127–31, 135–36; unilateral, 122. *See also specific procedures*

breast reduction as risk modifier, 30–31

breast self-exams (BSE), 78–79, 114, 196, 209

breast surgeon, 116

breast symmetry, 116, 122, 134

buproprion (Wellbutrin), 96, 153

CA-125 blood test, 84*t*, 85–86, 91, 222

calcitonin, 159

cancer: colon, 40, 90, 161, 174; endometrial, 40, 97; esophageal, 91, 102, 159; fallopian tube, 10–11, 23, 37, 55, 90–91, 138–39, 142–43, 187, 202; kidney, 40, 179; leukemia, 41; lung, 4–5, 202; lymphoma, 41, 124; melanoma, 12, 37, 40, 42, 92, 180, 206*t*, 214; pancreatic, 11–12, 23, 37, 42, 91, 174, 206*t*, 214, 219–20; peritoneal, 10–11, 23, 90–91, 138*t*, 139, 142, 187; prostate, 13, 23, 37, 92, 174, 206*t*, 211–14, 219–20; stomach, 91; uterine, 39, 91, 96–98, 143, 152, 160–61, 199. *See also* breast cancer, overview; ovarian cancer, overview

Cancer Information Service (NCI), 217

cancer statistics: average risk for BRCA mutation carriers, 33, 34*t*; breast cancer in U.S., 3–4, 5*t*, 25–26, 217; international cancer rates, 170; lifetime risk as percentage, 31–33; male breast cancer, 207; in media reports, 34; ovarian cancer in U.S., 9*t*, 25; young women with breast cancer, 195

capsular contracture, 127

carboplatin, 218–19

Celebrex, 100

Celexa, 96

cellular function, 17–22, 102–3, 169, 218–20

chemoprevention for breast cancer, 94–103; aromatase inhibitors, 98–99; bisphosphonates, 101–2; comparison of risk-reducing methods, 232*t*; deslorelin, 101; fenretinide, 100–101; and insurance and payment issues, 104–5; metformin, 102; nonsteroidal anti-inflammatory drugs, 99–100, 104; PARP

chemoprevention for breast cancer, *(cont.)*
inhibitors, 219–20; raloxifene, 95–97; tamoxifen, 95–97

chemoprevention for ovarian cancer, 103–5; analgesics, 104; comparison of risk-reducing methods, 232*t*; fenretinide, 104; and insurance and payment issues, 104–5; oral contraceptives, 103–4, 198

chemotherapy: adjuvant, 115, 218; and delay of reconstruction, 121–22; for hereditary cancers, 218–20; impact on survival, 231; for male breast cancer, 210; menopause due to, 196; neoadjuvant, 218–19; postlumpectomy, 115; for prostate cancer, 212

children: and adoption, 202; discussing cancer with, 61, 189–91; and genetic testing issues, 61; and odds of inheriting BRCA mutation, 36–38

chromosomes, 16

cisplatin, 218–19

City of Hope, 62

clinical breast exam (CBE), 78*t*, 79, 209

clinical trials, 224. *See also specific trials*

clomiphene citrate (Clomid), 199

collagen, 156

colon cancer, 40, 90, 161, 174. *See also* Lynch syndrome

colonoscopy, 39, 90

Community Living Assistance Services and Supports Act, 225

compounded hormones, 162–64

computed tomography (CT), 90

contralateral prophylactic mastectomy, 115–16

Coumadin, 154

Cowden syndrome, 40

cryosurgery, 212

culture and perception of risk, 31

DCIS. *See* ductal carcinoma in situ (DCIS)

decision making, 228–36; and breast cancer risk, 231; comparison of risk-reducing methods, 232*t*; comparison of treatments, 233–34; and genetic testing, 228–29; and risk reduction, 229–33; steps for, 234–35; and survival probability, 229–31; and treatment, 233–34

deep inferior epigastric perforator (DIEP) flap, 129, 135–36

deleterious mutation, 67

dense breasts, 29, 83, 101, 195–96

depression. *See* emotional issues

dermatologist, 92

deslorelin, 101

diet and nutrition: antioxidant properties of, 171; Asian diet, 172, 174; and breast cancer risk, 170–76; and dairy products, 173; effect on weight control, 174–76; and fish oil, 174; during menopause, 156; nutrigenomics, 177; and omega-3 fatty acids, 174; and prostate cancer risk, 213; during recovery, 130; and salmon, 174, 213; and soy food products, 172–73; studies on, 169–73

digital mammography, 80, 89, 180

digital rectal exams, 211–12

digital tomosynthesis, 83–84

diindolymethane (DIM), 174

direct-to-implant reconstruction, 125–26, 136

disability insurance, 225

DNA (deoxyribonucleic acid), 16–22, 62

DNA banking, 62

dong quai, 151

double mutations, 37

drug interactions, 96

dual-energy x-ray absorptiometry (DEXA), 158

ductal carcinoma in situ (DCIS), 6–7, 83, 95–96, 100–102; in men, 209

Duke University, 79

Effexor, 96, 152

embryo screening, 199, 204

emotional issues, 72–73, 96, 154–55, 197, 203

endocrinologist, 158

endometrial biopsy, 91

endometrial cancer, 40, 97

environmental exposure, 22, 69, 180–81

epigenetics, 177

esophageal cancer, 91, 102, 159

estriol, 162

estrogen, 7–9, 30, 94, 104, 153, 175

estrogen receptor–negative (ER–) tumors, 8, 95–96, 218

estrogen receptor–positive (ER+) tumors, 7–8; AI treatment, 98; chemoprevention, 232*t*; metformin trials, 102; phytoestrogens, effect of, 172; recurrence after oophorectomy, 147; risks of hormone replacement therapy, 163; tamoxifen, 95, 97, 210; testing for likelihood of recurrence, 218

estrogen replacement therapy (ERT), 143, 152, 157–60, 179

Evista. *See* raloxifene

exercise. *See* physical activity

expanders, 122, 124–25, 131*t*

Facing Our Risk of Cancer Empowered (FORCE): and free testing resources, 63; helpline of, 235; and information sharing worksheet, 184*t*; and male study volunteers, 215; and men's support groups, 216; message boards of, 120; outreach groups of, 235; website of, 46

Factor V Leiden mutation, 97

fallopian tube cancer, 10–11, 23, 37, 55, 90–91, 138–39, 142–43, 187, 202

fallopian tubes, 8, 38, 87; as origin of ovarian cancer, 87, 142; removal of, 138–43, 161; and tubal ligation, 30, 145, 198

family, sharing genetic testing results with, 183–88

family medical history: creating, 42–46; and diet, 170–71; and hidden risk, 37–38; and pedigree, 42; relatives, defined, 42–43; and risk factors for breast and ovarian cancer, 28–29. *See also* information sharing; pedigree

family planning, 198–202, 212

fanconi anemia (FA), 37

fareston, 94

fatigue, 10, 37, 139–40, 154–55, 212, 218

FDA. *See* U.S. Food and Drug Administration (FDA)

female reproductive system, 8–9

fenretinide, 100–101, 104

fertility, 139, 150–51, 154, 197–99

fertility specialists, 199

foods. *See* diet and nutrition

FORCE. *See* Facing Our Risk of Cancer Empowered (FORCE)

Forteo, 159

Fosamax, 102, 159

founder mutations, 23, 69

free flap reconstruction, 129

Gail Model, 22, 27–28, 96

gall bladder disease, 160

GAP flap reconstruction, 130, 136

genes and genetics: and cell division, 17, 19–20; and damage control process, 20–21; and diet, 172, 177; and DNA structure, 16–22, 62; and mutations, 3, 18–22; and proteins, 18; rearrangements, 19; study of, 14–16; and tumor-

genes and genetics: and cell division, *(cont.)*
  suppressor genes, 22. *See also* hereditary cancer syndromes
genes linked to breast cancer: ATM genes, 21; BRIP1 genes, 21; CDKN2A genes, 42; CHEK2 genes, 21; PALB2 genes, 21; PTEN genes, 21, 40; STK11 genes, 21, 41; TP53 genes, 21, 40. *See also* BRCA1 gene mutation, overview; BRCA2 gene mutation, overview
genetic counseling, 49–57, 62; benefits of, 49–50, 229; expertise, 52–54; identifying family members for testing, 54–55, 187; and insurance and payment issues, 56, 148; for men, 206; questions for counselor, 55
genetic discrimination, 63–65, 192
Genetic Information Nondiscrimination Act (GINA), 63–65, 192
genetic testing, 58–74; accuracy of, 71; advantages and disadvantages of, 58, 60; of children, 61; costs of, 59; and emotional issues, 72–73; and genetic variants, 70–71; GINA, discrimination protections, 63–65; and insurance and payment issues, 60, 63–65, 214–15; referral process for, 50–52; and sharing information with family, 183–88; and treatment choices, 61–65; and types of tests, 58–60; without genetic counseling, 51, 56
genetic test results: negative, 68–69, 72; no mutation detected, 68–69; positive, 67–68, 71; variant of uncertain significance, 70–71
genital fibroids, 40
Georgetown University Medical Center, 171
ginkgo biloba, 156
ginseng, 151

glucosamine, 156
gonadotropin inhibitors, 210
gynecologic oncologist, 90, 141
gynecologic surgeries, 138–49; and bone density tests, 158; and breast cancer survivor issues, 147–48; in combination with mastectomy, 145–47, 147t; and high-risk young women, 202; hysterectomy, 143–45, 147–48, 160–61, 164, 199, 202, 230-31, 232t, 233t; and insurance and payment issues, 148; oophorectomy, 138–44, 147t, 160–61, 164, 196–97, 202, 221t, 230-33, 233t; as risk reduction strategy, 145–47; tubal ligation, 145. *See also specific types*
gynecologist, 141
gynecomastia, 208

HABITS trial, 163
Halsted radical mastectomy, 107
Harvard University, 79
HealthCare.gov, 225
health insurance and payment issues: and bone density tests, 164; and breast prostheses, 135; and breast reconstruction, 135–37; and cancer screening, 92–93; and clinical trials, 104–5, 225; and compounded hormones, 164; and genetic counseling, 56; and genetic testing, 60, 63–65, 214–15; and gynecologic surgeries, 148; and hereditary cancer, 224–25; and high-risk young women, 204; and mastectomy, 119, 135; and men and BRCA, 214–15; and pre-existing conditions, 64–65; and preimplantation genetic diagnosis, 204; and preventive oophorectomy, 148; and prophylactic hysterectomy, 148; and PSA testing, 215; and saliva testing for hormones, 164; and in vitro fertilization, 204

Health Insurance Portability and Accountability Act (HIPAA), 64
healthy diet. *See* diet and nutrition
heart disease, 26, 100, 150, 157–58, 161, 170–71, 202
hematoma, 117
HER2, 8, 210
herbal supplements, 151–52, 154, 156, 162
Herceptin, 210
hereditary breast and ovarian cancer (HBOC) syndrome, 38–39, 136
hereditary cancer, diagnosis and treatment, 217–27; breast cancer issues, 208–10, 220–21; chemotherapy, 218–19; clinical trials, 224; insurance and payment issues, 224–25; ovarian cancer issues, 222–23; PARP inhibitors, 219–20; prostate cancer, 13, 23, 37, 92, 206*t*, 211–14, 219–20; second opinions, 217; treatment methods, 218–20; tumor gene assessment, 218. *See also specific types*
hereditary cancer syndromes, 36–46; ataxia-telangiectasia, 41; Cowden syndrome, 40; HBOC syndrome, 38–39, 136; hereditary diffuse gastric cancer, 41; Li-Fraumeni syndrome, 40–41; Lynch syndrome, 39–40, 90–91, 143; Peutz-Jeghers syndrome, 41
hereditary diffuse gastric cancer, 41
hereditary nonpolyposis colorectal cancer (HNPCC). *See* Lynch syndrome
hernia, 129
high-grade serous ovarian tumor, 85
Hispanic Americans, risk and cancer rates, 23, 29
hormone receptor–negative, 198
hormone receptors, defined, 7
hormone replacement therapy: bioidenticals, 162; and breast cancer risk, 30, 160 61; and compounded hormones, 162–63; contraindications for, 197;

and hysterectomy, 143; and low-dose estrogen skin patch, 160; for men, 212; and menopause, 158–64; and ovarian cancer risk, 160
hot flashes, 151–52
Human Genome Project, 15
hydration before surgery, 130
hysterectomy, 143–45, 147–48, 160–61, 164, 199, 202

immune system, 109, 122, 131, 174
IMPACT study, 212, 215
implants. *See* breast implants
infection, 37, 127, 159, 179; after surgery, 109, 117–18, 121–24, 130, 133*t*, 142*t*, 144
inferior gluteal artery perforator (IGAP) flap, 130, 136
infertility, 29
inflammatory breast cancer (IBC), 7, 209
information sharing, 183–93; with children, 189–91; discussing genetic testing with family, 183–88; GINA protections, 192; male reactions of avoidance/denial, 207; and nonsupportive people, 191; with partners, 188–91; sexuality and sensuality, 188–90; with spouses, 188–91; when dating, 189–90; in workplace, 191–92; worksheet, 184*t*
inherited mutations, 20, 36–37
in situ breast tumors, 6–7
insomnia, menopausal, 153–54
insurance. *See* health insurance and payment issues
integrative oncology, 177
International Agency for Research on Cancer, 176, 180
invasive breast tumors, 6–7
invasive ductal carcinoma (IDC), 6, 209
invasive lobular carcinoma (ILC), 6–7, 209
in vitro fertilization, 147*t*, 199, 204, 214

Johns Hopkins University, meta-analysis, 33, 34*t*
joint pain, menopausal, 156

kava, 154
kidney cancer, 40, 179
King, Mary-Claire, 15
Klinefelter syndrome, 208

laparoscopically assisted vaginal hysterectomy (LAVH), 144
laparoscopic oophorectomy, 139–41, 144
laparotomy, 140–41
lateral transverse flap, 129
latissimus dorsi flap, 128–29
leukemia, 41
leuprolide acetate (Lupron), 196–97
Lexapro, 96, 152
libido. *See* sexual desire and intimacy
life insurance, 204
lifestyle choices and risk, 28, 169–82; alcohol consumption, 30, 178; environmental exposure, 180–81; hormone replacement therapy, 178–79; men and BRCA, 213–14; during menopause, 157–63; myths, 181; nutrition, 169–76; physical activity, 176–77; smoking, 179–80. *See also specific lifestyle choices*
lifetime risk: BRCA-related fallopian tube cancer, 11; BRCA-related primary peritoneal cancer, 11; breast cancer, 5, 28–29, 31–33, 41, 78, 113–14; melanoma, 42; men's risk for cancer, 206*t*, 211; ovarian cancer, 9*t*, 223; pancreatic cancer, 12, 42; as percentage, 31–33; primary peritoneal cancer, 139; prostate cancer, 211
Li-Fraumeni syndrome, 40–41
lignans, 172–73
limited family structure, defined, 62
lobular carcinoma in situ (LCIS), 6, 96

Locholest, 97
low-dose estrogen skin patch, 160
lumpectomy, 61, 114–15, 148, 210, 221*t*, 233*t*
lung cancer, 4–5, 202
Lupron, 196–97
lymphatic system, 109
lymphedema, 118–19
lymph node removal, 108–10, 117–18, 141
lymph nodes, 6–7, 109–10, 117, 141, 213
lymphoma, 41, 124
Lynch syndrome, 39–40, 90–91, 143

magnetic resonance imaging (MRI): comparison to mammograms, 83; and contralateral mastectomy, 116; and DCIS detection, 6, 83; as early detection strategy, 78*t*, 79, 82–83; and high-risk young women, 196; and insurance and payment issues, 92; postmastectomy, 114; of silicone implants, 124
male breast cancer, 207–10
MammaPrint test, 218
mammograms and mammography: after breast cancer, 82; comparison to MRI, 83; and DCIS detection, 6; and diagnosis, 5; digital procedures, 80; as early detection strategy, 78*t*, 79–82; and FDA-certified facilities, 82; and insurance and payment issues, 92; for men, 209; and radiation exposure, 81; for women over 65, 81; for women under 30, 81; for women under 40, 195–96
massage, 118, 177
mastectomy, 107–20; areola-sparing, 113–14; bilateral, 61–62, 69, 82, 107, 221*t*, 233*t*; as breast cancer treatment, 114–16, 209–10; and breast surgeon, 116; in combination with oophorectomy, 145–47, 147*t*; comparison of risk-reducing methods, 232*t*; contralateral prophylactic, 115–16; and immediate

reconstruction, 108–10; and insurance and payment issues, 119; modified radical, 108, 209–10; nipple-sparing, 111–13, 126; and postmastectomy pain syndrome, 117–18; during pregnancy, 199–200; prophylactic, 107–10, 113–14, 121, 126, 161, 222, 230, 233*t*; radical, 107–8, 209–10; risk and recovery, 116–18; and sensation after surgery, 108; seroma, 117; skin-sparing procedures, 110–14, 117*t*; subcutaneous, 113; and survival probability, 231; total, 108, 209–10; unilateral, 107, 122–23, 148, 221*t*, 233*t*; without reconstruction, 123

Mayo Clinic, 157–58

Medicaid, 92, 225

Medicare, 63, 92, 225

Megace, 210

melanoma, 12, 37, 40, 42, 92, 180, 206*t*, 214

melatonin, 180

memory changes, menopausal, 156

men and BRCA, 206–16; cancer risk comparisons, 38, 206*t*; FORCE support groups, 216; and insurance and payment issues, 214–15; and male breast cancer, 207–10; and preimplantation genetic diagnosis, 212; and prostate cancer risk, 211–14; reaction to risk, 207; and risk of other hereditary cancers, 214–15; and screening and treatment, 208–10; and in vitro fertilization, 212

menarche onset age, 29

Mendel, Gregor, 14

menopause, 150–65; and breast cancer survivor issues, 163; caused by chemotherapy, 196; caused by oophorectomy, 151; and heart disease risk, 157–58; and insurance and payment issues, 164; and ovaries, 9; perimenopause, 150–51; premature, 150

menopause symptoms: bone loss, 158–59; decreased libido, 152–53; depression, 154–55; fatigue, 154; hormone replacement therapy for, 159–64; hot flashes, 151–52; joint pain, 156; memory changes, 156; mood swings, 154–55; night sweats, 151, 153; skin and hair changes, 156; sleep disturbances, 153–54, 156; urinary problems, 157; vaginal dryness/atrophy, 152; weight gain, 152, 155

mental health professionals, 154–55

message boards, FORCE, 120

metastasize, defined, 6–7

metformin, 102

microcalcifications, 6, 80, 83, 89

microwave ovens and risk, 181

molecular breast imaging, 84

MRI. *See* magnetic resonance imaging (MRI)

muscle loss, 129, 134, 176–77

mutations: acquired vs. inherited, 20; BRCA founder mutations, 23, 69; as cause of breast and ovarian cancers, 3; explanation of, 18–23; rearrangements, 19. *See also specific mutations*

My Family Health Portrait, 45

Myriad Genetics, 58–60, 63

National Breast and Cervical Cancer Early Detection Program, 93

National Cancer Institute (NCI), 26, 80, 217

National Comprehensive Cancer Network (NCCN) recommendations: and breast cancer surveillance, 78*t*; and contralateral mastectomy, 115–16; and genetic counseling and testing, 50–51, 195; and mammograms for high-risk young women, 81; and ovarian cancer surveillance, 84*t*; and prostate cancer screening, 211–12

National Gene Test Fund, 63

National Institutes of Health, 138

necrosis, 122, 128

needle aspiration, 88, 213

needle biopsy, 88

negative test results, 68–69, 72

neoadjuvant chemotherapy, 218–19

nicotine, 130

night-shift work, 180

night sweats, 151, 153

nighttime exposure to artificial light, 180

nipple reconstruction, 121, 126, 131–34, 132*f*

nipple-sparing mastectomy, 111–13, 126

no mutation detected, test result, 68–69

nonexpansive implant reconstruction, 125–26, 136

non-hereditary cancer, incidence of, 3–4. *See also* sporadic cancer

nonsteroidal anti-inflammatory drugs (NSAIDs), 99–100, 104, 156

North American Menopause Society (NAMS), 162–63

nucleus, 16–17

Nurses' Health Study, 100, 104

nutrigenomics, 177

nutrition. *See* diet and nutrition

obesity, 30, 130, 174–75

oncologist, 7, 109, 197–99, 213

OncoType DX, 218

one-step reconstruction, 125–26, 136

oophorectomy, 138–48, 197, 221*t*, 230; abdominal wash, 140–41; comparison of risk-reducing methods, 221*t*, 232*t*; defined, 138; for high-risk young women, 196–97, 202; hormone replacement therapy after, 160–61, 164; and insurance and payment issues, 148; with laparoscopically assisted vaginal hysterectomy, 144; laparoscopic BSO, 139–41, 144; laparotomy,

140–41; mastectomy in combination with, 145–47, 147*t*; prophylactic bilateral salpingo-oophorectomy (BSO), 86–88, 138–44, 146, 147*t*, 160–61, 164, 197, 202, 232–33*t*; recovery, 140; risk of breast cancer recurrence after, 147; robotic surgery, 144; survival probability, 230–31

ophthalmologist, 92, 214

oral contraceptives, 30, 198, 232; comparison of risk-reducing methods, 232*t*

osteonecrosis of jaw, 159

osteoporosis, 101–2, 158–59

ostopenia, 158

OVA1 blood test, 90

ovarian cancer, overview, 8–11; BRCA1 and BRCA2, 3–4; and breast cancer risk, 222; chemotherapy for, 218–19; detection of, 9; exploratory surgery for, 90; incidence of, 3–4, 9*t*; origin in fallopian tubes, 87, 142; PARP inhibitors for, 219–20; and pregnancy, 200–201; and related cancers, 10–11; surveillance for, 84–88; survival rates, 222; symptoms of, 10; treatment, 218–20

ovarian cancer risk: for average women, 9, 25; after breast cancer, 223; lifetime risk with BRCA mutation, 32–34; and risk factors, 28–31

ovaries, description and function of, 8–9

Paget's disease, 7

pain specialists, 118

pancreatic cancer, 11–12, 23, 37, 42, 91, 174, 206*t*, 214, 219–20

Pap smears, 84, 152

parabens, 181

parathyroid hormone (PTH), 159

PARP inhibitors (PARPis), 102–3, 212–13, 219–20

pathology, 141, 209

Patient Protection and Affordable Care Act (2010), 64–65, 92, 224–25

Paxil, 96, 152

payment assistance, 63, 136, 218. *See also* health insurance and payment issues

PBM. *See* prophylactic bilateral mastectomy (PBM)

pedigree, 42–46, 51, 54–56, 70–71. *See also* family medical history

pelvic exams, 84*f*, 85, 91

pelvic floor conditioning, 157

perforator flap reconstruction, 129–30

perimenopause, 150–51

peritoneal cancer. *See* primary peritoneal cancer

peritoneal wash, 141

Peutz-Jeghers syndrome, 41

physical activity: to build bones, 158; and menopausal symptoms, 151–55; and reconstruction recovery, 131; as risk modifier, 30, 176–77; yoga, 118, 151, 155

physical therapist, 118

physical therapy, 118, 156

phytochemicals, 171–72

phytoestrogens, 172–73

plastic surgeon, 121, 124, 134–37

platinum drugs, 218–19

positive for a deleterious mutation, defined, 67

positive self-talk, 190

positive test results, 67–68, 71

positron emission mammography, 84

postmastectomy pain syndrome (PMPS), 117–18

Pre-Existing Condition Insurance Plan program, 65

pre-existing conditions, 64–65

pregnancy, 30, 199–201

preimplantation genetic diagnosis (PGD), 199, 204, 212, 214

Premarin, 160

premenopausal diagnosis, 196–98

Prevention and Observation of Surgical Endpoints (PROSE), 138, 202

previvors: and alcohol consumption, 164; defined, 12; and hormone replacement therapy, 30, 160–61, 164, 179, 202; tamoxifen for, 95–96, 105; young, 194–95. *See also specific diagnoses and treatments*

primary peritoneal cancer, 10–11, 23, 90–91, 138*t*, 139, 142, 187

privacy rights, 64–65

progesterone, 9

progesterone creams, 152

progesterone receptor–negative (PR–) tumors, 8, 218

progesterone receptor–positive (PR+) tumors, 7–8, 98, 147, 218, 232*t*; recurrence after oophorectomy, 147

progestin, 161

prophylactic bilateral mastectomy (PBM), 107–10, 113–14, 121, 126, 161, 222, 233*t*. *See also* mastectomy

prophylactic bilateral salpingo-oophorectomy (BSO), 86–88, 138–44, 146, 147*t*, 160–61, 164, 197, 202, 232–33*t*. *See also* oophorectomy

prostate cancer, 13, 23, 37, 92, 174, 206*t*, 211–14, 219–20

prostatectomy, 212

prostate-specific antigen (PSA) blood test, 211

proteins, 18

Prozac, 96, 152

questions to ask: breast surgeons about mastectomy, 116; genetic counselors, 55; gynecologic surgeons, 140; MRI facilities, 83; plastic surgeons about reconstruction, 126, 135

Questran, 97

race and ethnicity, risk and cancer rates, 7, 23, 29, 37. *See also specific groups*

radiation exposure, 29, 81, 180

radiation treatments, 114–15, 200, 212, 221*t*, 231, 233*t*; and reconstruction, 121–22

raloxifene, 94, 96–97, 105, 159

rearrangements, 19, 59

receptor-negative (ER– and PR–) tumors, 8, 95–96, 218

Reclast, 159

reconstruction. *See* breast reconstruction

recovery: from hysterectomy, 144; from mastectomy, 116; from oophorectomy, 140; from reconstructive surgery, 121, 124–26, 129–34

rectovaginal exam, 85

recurrence: of breast cancer, 6, 95, 98, 104, 114, 147, 163; of ER+ tumors after oophorectomy, 147; of ovarian cancer, 219; of PR+ tumors after oophorectomy, 147; and pregnancy-related breast cancer, 200; and testing approaches, 218

red clover, 151

relative risk, defined, 32

relatives. *See* family medical history; information sharing

resources: BRCA and men, 216; breast cancer, 13, 35; breast reconstruction, 125, 137; cancer risk, 35; chemoprevention, 106; diagnosis of hereditary cancer, 227; early detection, 93; genetic counseling, 57; genetics, 24; genetic testing, 66, 74; gynecologic surgeries, 149; hereditary cancer risk, 46; high-risk young women, 205; information sharing, 193; lifestyle choices, 182; mastectomy, 120; menopause, 165; oophorectomy, 149; ovarian cancer, 13, 35

risk, overview, 25–35; absolute, 31–32; average, 25, 33, 34*t*; calculation of, 31–34; incremental, 33; inherited, 11, 87, 169, 184; lifetime, 31–33; relative, 32. *See also* cancer statistics

risk assessment: and Asian women, 52; and Gail Model, 27; and risk factors, 28–31. *See also* genetic counseling

risk management: for breast cancer, 77–84; for ovarian cancer, 84–88. *See also* risk reduction

risk reduction: chemoprevention and, 94–106; and contralateral breast cancer, 115–16; and lifestyle choices, 169–82; making decisions about, 229–33; and prophylactic bilateral mastectomy (PBM), 107–10, 113–14, 121, 126, 161, 222, 233*t*; and prophylactic bilateral salpingo-oophorectomy (BSO), 86–88, 138–44, 146, 147*t*, 160–61, 164, 197, 202, 232–33*t*

risk statistics, 26–28

robotic surgery, 144

saline breast implants, 122, 124–27

sampling lymph nodes, 109–10, 118, 210; and risk of lymphedema, 118–19

screening for cancer. *See* surveillance for breast cancer; surveillance for other cancers; surveillance for ovarian cancer

second opinions, 10, 135, 217

selective estrogen receptor modulators (SERMs), 94–97

selective serotonin reuptake inhibitors (SSRIs), 96, 152

sensation, after mastectomy, 108, 132

sensitivity in screening tests, 77–78

sentinel node biopsy, 109–10, 210

Sephardic Jews, 59

serial sectioning of ovaries and tubes, 141

seroma, 117

sexual desire and intimacy, 152–53, 188–90

silicone breast implants, 124–27

silicone prostheses, 123

single-nucleotide polymorphisms (SNPs), 21–22

single-stage reconstruction, 125–26, 136

skin and hair changes, menopausal, 156

skin-sparing mastectomy, 110*f*, 110–14, 111*f*

sleep disturbances, menopausal, 153–54, 156

smoking, 12, 20, 28, 130–31, 156–57, 179–80

Social Security disability benefits, 225

Society of Gynecologic Oncologists, 141

sonograms, 89

soy and breast cancer risk, 172

specificity in screening tests, 78

sporadic breast cancer, 3–4, 61–62, 98, 104, 115–16, 175–76, 201. *See also* breast cancer, overview

sporadic cancer, 3–4, 51

sporadic ovarian cancer, 142, 222

SSRIs, 96, 152

staging cancers, 7, 109

Stanford University survival model, 229

state laws: about genetic discrimination, 64; about reconstruction, 137

statins, 101

stereotactic biopsy, 89

St. John's wort, 154

stomach cancer, 91

stress-management techniques, 151

Study of Tamoxifen and Raloxifene (STAR) trial, 96

subcutaneous mastectomy, 113

submammary mastectomy, 113

sunlight, 174

superficial inferior epigastric artery perforator (SIEA) flap, 129–30

superior gluteal artery perforator (SGAP) flap, 130, 136

supplements. *See* herbal supplements; vitamins and supplements

surgical biopsy, 89

surgical complications: of mastectomy, 116–17; of oophorectomy, 142; of reconstruction, 133–34

surgical drains, 118

surgical menopause. *See* menopause

surgical risks with mastectomy, 116–18, 117*t*

surveillance for breast cancer, 77–84; breast biopsy, 6, 82–84, 88–89, 209; breast self-exams, 78–79, 114, 196, 209; breast ultrasound, 89, 209; clinical breast exams, 78*t*, 79, 209; comparison of risk-reducing methods, 232*t*; digital tomosynthesis, 83–84; insurance and payment issues, 92–93; mammograms, 78, 79–82; molecular breast imaging, 84; MRI screening, 78*t*, 79, 82–83; NCCN screening recommendations, 78*t*, 195; positron emission mammography, 84

surveillance for other cancers: colon, 90; esophageal, 91; fallopian tube, 90–91; melanoma, 92; pancreatic, 91; primary peritoneal, 90–91; prostate, 92, 211–12; stomach, 91; uterine, 91

surveillance for ovarian cancer, 84–88; biomarkers, 86–87; CA-125 blood test, 84*t*, 85–86, 91, 222; NCCN screening recommendations, 84*t*; pelvic exams, 84*t*, 85, 91; transvaginal ultrasound with color Doppler, 84*t*, 85–86, 91

survivor, defined, 12

Susan G. Komen for the Cure, 79, 119

tamoxifen, 94–97, 99, 105, 143, 147, 210

tattooing nipples and areolas, 121, 132

teriparatide (Forteo), 159

testicles, 212

testosterone, 153

test results, 68–69, 71–73. *See also specific tests*

tests for cancer. *See* surveillance for breast cancer; surveillance for other cancers; surveillance for ovarian cancer

thyroid problems, 154

tissue flap reconstruction: attached flaps, 128–29; challenges of, 127–28; and chemotherapy, 122; comparison of techniques, 131*t*; free flap, 129; and insurance and payment issues, 135; perforator flaps, 129–30; and radiation, 122. *See also specific types*

total abdominal hysterectomy with BSO (TAH/BSO), 144

transverse rectus abdominis myocutaneous (TRAM) flap, 128–29

transverse upper gracilis (TUG) flap, 129

trastuzumab (Herceptin), 210

treatments. *See specific treatments*

tubal hypothesis, 142

tubal ligation, 30, 145, 198

tumor: breast cancer, 6–8, 21, 95–96, 100–101; gene testing of, 218; ovarian cancer, 85; and staging cancers, 7; tumor-suppressor genes, 22. *See also specific types*

type 2 diabetes, 102

ultrasound: breast, 89, 209; endoscopic, 91; transvaginal, with color Doppler, 84*t*, 85–86, 91

underwire bras and breast cancer risk, 181

unilateral breast reconstruction, 122

unilateral mastectomy. *See* mastectomy

uninformative tests, use of term, 70

University of Washington, 142

urethral sphincters, 157

urinary problems, menopausal, 157

U.S. Food and Drug Administration (FDA): bioidentical hormones, 162; compounded hormones, 162; ERT approval, 152; herbal preparations, 152, 162; mammography facility database, 82; MRI screening of silicone implants, 124; study on BPA, 181; study on parabens, 181

U.S. Health and Human Services Department, 45

uterine cancer, 39, 91, 96–98, 143, 152, 160–61, 199

uterine fibroid, 40, 86, 143

uterus, 8–9, 85, 97, 143–45, 152, 160–61, 199

vaginal bleeding, 11, 91, 97, 143

vaginal dryness/atrophy, menopausal, 152

vaginal estrogen creams, 197–98

vaginal exams, 84–85, 152

vaginal ultrasound, 84*t*, 85–86, 91

valerian, 154

variant of uncertain significance (VUS), 70–71

virtual colonoscopy, 90

vision exams, 92

vitamins and supplements, 40, 152, 156, 158–59, 173–74. *See also* herbal supplements

weight control, 152, 155, 174–76. *See also* physical activity

Wellbutrin, 96, 153

Women's Health and Cancer Rights Act (WHCRA), 135

Women's Health Initiative, 99–102, 155, 161

yoga, 118, 151, 155
young women at high risk, 194–205;
    and adoption, 202; and birth control,
    198; and breast cancer and pregnancy,
    199–200; and breastfeeding, 198–201;
    and diagnostic difficulties, 195–96;
    emotional issues of, 197, 203; and
    family planning, 198–202; fertility of,
    197–99; genetic testing of, 194–95; and
insurance and payment issues, 204;
parity of, 200–201; and preimplantation genetic diagnosis (PGD), 199;
and premenopause diagnoses, 196–98;
and salpingo-oophorectomy, 202; and
in vitro fertilization, 199; and young
menopause, 197–98

Zoladex, 196–97

About the Authors

SUE FRIEDMAN, D.V.M., gave up her career as a veterinarian to found Facing Our Risk of Cancer Empowered (FORCE), the only national organization dedicated to improving the lives of individuals at high risk for inherited breast and ovarian cancer. Under her direction, FORCE has educated hundreds of thousands of people about the latest advances in cancer prevention, detection, treatment, and related quality-of-life issues. A breast cancer survivor, Sue lives in Florida.

REBECCA SUTPHEN, M.D., F.A.C.M.G., is a board-certified clinical and molecular geneticist with clinical and research expertise in hereditary cancer. She served as director of clinical genetics at Moffitt Cancer Center at the University of South Florida from the program's founding in 1996 until 2009, when she accepted a new role to promote telephone access to board-certified genetics experts as chief medical officer for the country's largest independent genetic counseling provider, Informed Medical Decisions. She continues her research as a professor in the USF College of Medicine. Rebecca is a member of FORCE's Board of Directors and Medical Advisory Board. A breast cancer survivor, Rebecca lives in Florida.

KATHY STELIGO is a freelance business and health writer. She is the author of *The Breast Reconstruction Guidebook* and is editor-at-large for FORCE. A two-time breast cancer survivor, Kathy lives in California.